Advanced Health Assessment Technology

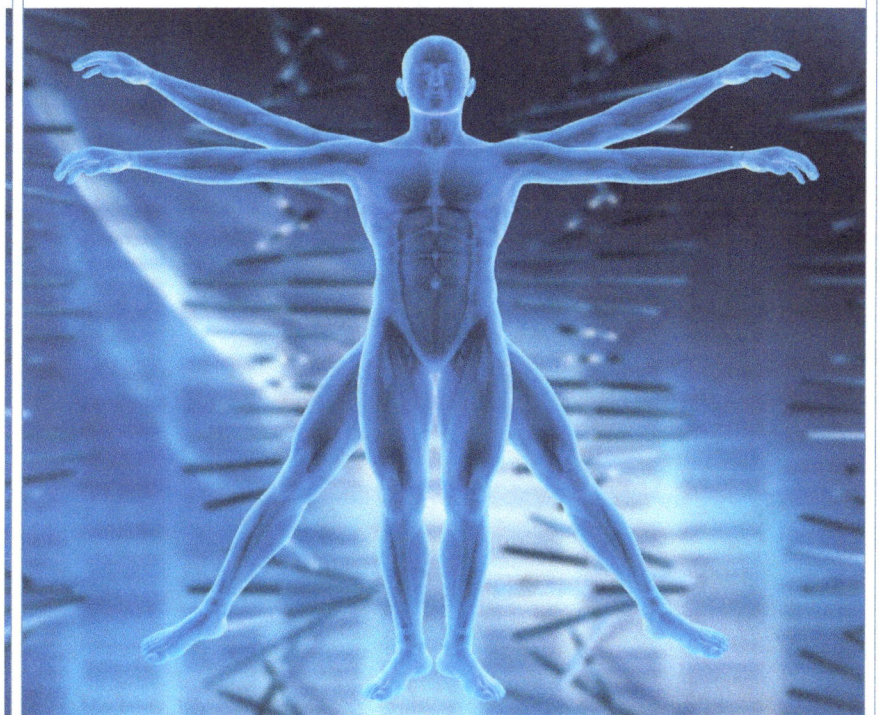

MEDICAL TERMINOLOGY

AUTHOR
EVELIN L KHOLELI

Table of Content

1. Cardiovascular and Cerebrovascular
- Blood viscosity
- Cholesterol Crystal
- Blood fat
- Vascular Resistance
- Vascular Elasticity
- Myocardial Blood Demand
- Myocardial Blood Perfusion Volume
- Myocardial Oxygen Consumption
- Stroke Volume
- Left Ventricular Ejection Impendence
- Left Ventricular Effective Pump Power
- Coronary Artery Elasticity
- Coronary Perfusion Pressure
- Cerebral Blood Vessel Elasticity
- Brain Tissue Blood Supply Status

2. Gastrointestinal function
- Pepsin Secretion Coefficient
- Gastric Peristalsis Function Coefficient
- Gastric Absorption Function Coefficient
- Small Intestine Peristalsis Function Coefficient
- Small Intestine Absorption Function Coefficient

3. Large Intestine Function
- Large Intestine Peristalsis Function Coefficient
- Colonic Absorption Coefficient
- Intestinal Bacteria Coefficient
- Intraluminal Pressure Coefficient

4. Liver Function
- Protein Metabolism
- Energy Production Function
- Detoxification Function
- Bile Secretion Function
- Liver Fat Content

5. Gallbladder Function
- Serum Globulin
- Total Bilirubin
- Alkaline Phosphatase
- Serum Total Bile Acid
- Bilirubin

6. Pancreatic Function
- Insulin
- Pancreatic Polypeptide
- Glucagon

7. Kidney Function
- Urobilinogen Index
- Uric Acid Index
- Blood Urea Nitrogen (BUN) Index
- Proteinuria Index

8. Lung Function
- Vital Capacity
- Total Lung Capacity
- Airway Resistance
- Arterial Oxygen Content

9. Brain Nerve
- Status of Brain Tissue Blood Supply

- Cerebral Arteriosclerosis
- Functional Status of Cranial Nerve
- Sentiment Index
- Memory Index

10. Bone Disease
11. Bone Mineral Density
- Osteoclast Coefficient
- Amount of Calcium Loss
- Degree of Bone Hyperplasia
- Degree of Osteoporosis
- Bone Mineral Density

12. Rheumatoid Bone Disease
- Degree of Cervical Calcification
- Degree of Lumbar Calcification
- Bone Hyperplasia Coefficient
- Osteoporosis Coefficient
- Rheumatism Coefficient

13. Bone Growth Index
- Bone Alkaline Phosphatase
- Osteocalcin
- Status of Long Bone Healing
- Short Bone Cartilage Healing Situation
- Epiphyseal Line

14. Blood Sugar
- Coefficient of Insulin Secretion
- Blood Sugar Coefficient
- Urine Sugar Coefficient

15. **Trace Elements**
    - Calcium
    - Iron
    - Zinc
    - Selenium
    - Phosphorus
    - Potassium
    - Magnesium
    - Copper
    - Cobalt
    - Manganese
    - Iodine
    - Nickel
    - Fluorine
    - Molybolenum
    - Vanadium
    - Tin
    - Silicon
    - Strontium
    - Boron
16. **Vitamin**
    - Vitamin A
    - Vitamin B1
    - Vitamin B2
    - Vitamin B3
    - Vitamin B6
    - Vitamin B12
    - Vitamin C
    - Vitamin D3
    - Vitamin E
    - Vitamin K

17. Amino Acid
- Lysine
- Tryptophan
- Phenylalanine
- Methionine
- Threonine
- Isoleucine
- Leocine
- Valine
- Histidine
- Arginine

18. Coenzyme
- Nicotinamide
- Biotin
- Panthothenic Acid
- Folic Acid
- Coenzyme Q10
- Glutathione

19. Fatty Acid
- Linoleic Acid
- a-Linoleic Acid
- r-Linolenic Acid
- Arachidonic Acid

20. Endocrine System
- Thyroid Secretion Index
- Parathyroid Hormone Secretion Index
- Adrenal Gland Index
- Pituary Secretion Index
- Pineal Secretion Index

- Thymus Gland Secretion Index
- Gland Secretion Index

21. Immune System
- Lymph Node Index
- Tonsil Immune Index
- Bone Marrow Index
- Spleen Index
- Thymus Index
- Immunoglobulin Index
- Respiratory Immune Index
- Gastrointestinal Immune Index
- Mucosa Immune Index

22. Thyroid
- Free Thyroxine Index (FT4)
- Thyroglobulin
- Anti-thyroglobulin Antibodies
- Three Triiodothyronine (T3)

23. Human Toxin
- Stimulating Beverage
- Electromagnetic Radiation
- Tobacco / Nicotine
- Toxic Pesticide Residue

24. Heavy Metal
- Lead
- Mercury
- Cadmium
- Chromium
- Arsenic
- Antimony

- Thallium
- Aluminum

25. Basic Physical Quality
- Response Ability
- Mental Power
- Water Shortage
- Hypoxia
- PH

26. Allergy
- Drug Allergy Index
- Alcohol Allergy Index
- Pollen Allergy Index
- Injection Allergy Index
- Chemical Products Allergy Index
- Paint Allergy Index
- Dust Allergy Index
- Smoke Allergy Index
- Hair Dye Allergy Index
- Animal Fur Allergy Index
- Metal Jewellery Index
- Seafood Allergy Index
- Milk Allergy Index

27. Obesity
- Abnormal Lipid Metabolism Coefficient
- Brown Adipose Tissue Abnormalities Coefficient
- Hyperinsulinemia Coefficient
- Nucleus of the Hypothalamus Abnormal Coefficient
- Triglyceride Content of Abnormal Coefficient

28. **Skin**
    - Skin Free Radical Index
    - Skin Collagen Index
    - Skin Grease Index
    - Skin Immunity Index
    - Skin Moisture Index
    - Skin Moisture Loss
    - Skin Red Blood Trace Index
    - Skin Elasticity Index
    - Skin Melanin Index
    - Skin Horniness Index

29. **Eye**
    - Bags under the eyes
    - Collagen Eye Wrinkle
    - Dark Circles
    - Lymphatic Obstruction
    - Sagging
    - Edema
    - Eye Cell Activity
    - Visual Fatigue

30. **Collagen**
    - Eye
    - Tooth
    - Hair and Skin
    - Endocrine System
    - Circulatory System
    - Digestive System
    - Immune System
    - Motion System
    - Muscle Tissue

- Fat Metabolism
- Detoxification and Metabolism
- Reproductive System
- Nervous System
- Skeleton

31. Channel and Collaterals
- Hand Tai Yin Lung Meridian
- Hand Yang Ming Large Intestine Meridian
- Foot Tai Yin Lung Meridian
- Hand Shao Yin Heart Sutra
- Hand The Small Intestine by the Sun
- Foot Tai Yang Bladder Meridian
- Foot Jue Yin Liver Meridian
- Ren Channel
- Governor Meridian
- Vital Meridian
- Tai Mai

32. Pulse of Heart and Brain
- Stroke Index
- Stroke Volume
- Heart Peripheral Resistance
- Pulse Wave Coefficient
- Cerebrovascular Blood Oxygen Saturation
- Cerebrovascular Blood Oxygen Volume
- Cerebrovascular Blood Oxygen Pressure

33. Blood Lipids
- Blood Viscosity
- Total Cholesterol
- Triglyceride
- High Density Lipoprotein

- Low Density Lipoprotein
- Neutral Fat
- Circulating Immune Complex

34. Gynecology
- Female Hormone
- Gonadotropin
- Prolactin
- Progesterone
- Vaginitis Coefficient
- PID Coefficient
- Appendagitis Coefficient
- Cervicitis Coefficient
- Ovarian Cyst Coefficient

35. Breast
- Hyperplasia of Mammary Glands Coefficient
- Acute Mastitis Coefficient
- Chronic Mastitis Coefficient
- Endocrine Dyscrasia Coefficient
- Fibroadenoma of Breast Coefficient

36. Menstrual Cycle
- Beta Hormone
- Reflect Protein
- Fibrinogen
- Sedimentation Rate

37. Prostate
- Degree of Prostatic Hyperplasia
- Degree of Prostatic Calcification
- Prostatitis Syndrome

38. Male Sexual Function
- Testerone
- Gonadotropin
- Erection Transmitter

39. Sperm and Semen
- Semen Volume
- Liquefying Time
- Number of Sperms
- Sperm Motility Rate

CARDIOVASCULAR AND CEREBROVASCULAR

Blood viscosity refers to the thickness and stickiness of blood, which affects its flow through the blood vessels. It is primarily determined by the concentration of red blood cells and the presence of plasma proteins in the blood. Factors such as hematocrit (the proportion of blood that is made up of red blood cells), plasma proteins, temperature, and shear stress also influence blood viscosity.

Higher viscosity means that blood is thicker and flows more slowly, which can increase resistance to blood flow through the vessels. This increased resistance can lead to issues such as high blood pressure and decreased circulation.

Several medical conditions can affect blood viscosity, including dehydration, polycythemia (an increase in the number of red blood cells), and certain genetic disorders. Conversely, low blood viscosity can occur in conditions such as anemia, where there is a decreased number of red blood cells, or in conditions associated with decreased plasma protein concentration.

Doctors may measure blood viscosity as part of assessing a person's cardiovascular health, especially if they are at risk of conditions such as stroke or heart disease. Treatments for abnormal blood viscosity depend on the underlying cause and may include medications, lifestyle changes, or medical procedures.

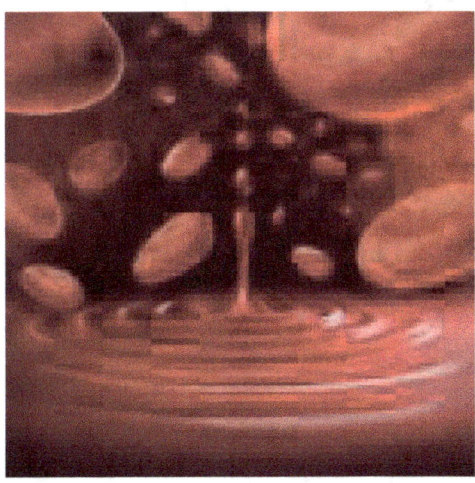

Cholesterol crystals are solid structures composed of cholesterol molecules. These crystals can form within the body, typically in the gallbladder, bile ducts, or within atherosclerotic plaques in blood vessels.

In the gallbladder, cholesterol crystals can contribute to the formation of gallstones, which are hardened deposits that can cause pain and other symptoms if they block the flow of bile.

In blood vessels, cholesterol crystals can be found within atherosclerotic plaques. Atherosclerosis is a condition characterized by the buildup of plaque, consisting of cholesterol, other lipids, calcium, and cellular debris, within the walls of arteries. The presence of cholesterol crystals within these plaques can trigger inflammation and lead to plaque rupture, which can result in the formation of blood clots and potentially lead to heart attacks or strokes.

Cholesterol crystals are a key component in the pathology of atherosclerosis and related cardiovascular diseases. Managing risk factors such as high cholesterol levels, hypertension, smoking, and diabetes can help reduce the risk of developing atherosclerosis and its complications. Additionally, medications such as statins may be prescribed to lower cholesterol levels and reduce the risk of plaque formation and cardiovascular events.

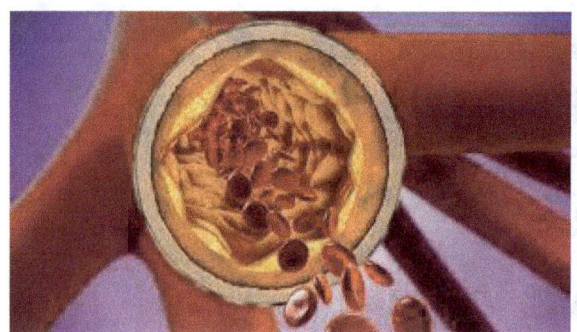

Blood fat is lipids, which are a type of fat found in the bloodstream. The main types of lipids found in the blood are triglycerides, cholesterol, and phospholipids. These lipids are carried in the bloodstream by lipoproteins, which are particles that consist of both lipids and proteins.

Here's a brief overview of these blood lipids:

- **Triglycerides**: These are the most common type of fat in the body and are primarily obtained from the diet. They are also synthesized by the liver. Elevated levels of triglycerides in the blood are associated with an increased risk of heart disease and other cardiovascular problems.

- **Cholestero**l: Cholesterol is a waxy, fat-like substance that is essential for building cell membranes and producing certain hormones. There are two main types of cholesterol: low-density lipoprotein (LDL) and high-density lipoprotein (HDL). LDL cholesterol is often referred to as "bad" cholesterol because high levels of it can lead to plaque buildup in the arteries, increasing the risk of heart disease. HDL cholesterol, on the other hand, is often called "good" cholesterol because it helps remove LDL cholesterol from the bloodstream, reducing the risk of heart disease.

- Phospholipids: These are another type of lipid found in the blood. They are essential components of cell membranes and are involved in various cellular processes.

Monitoring blood lipid levels, particularly triglycerides and cholesterol, is important for assessing cardiovascular health.

- High levels of triglycerides and LDL cholesterol, along with low levels of HDL cholesterol, are associated with an increased risk of heart disease and stroke. Lifestyle changes such as adopting a healthy diet, exercising regularly, and avoiding smoking can help improve blood lipid levels. In some cases, medications may also be prescribed to manage lipid levels.

Vascular resistance refers to the opposition that blood encounters as it flows through the blood vessels. It is a measure of how difficult it is for blood to flow through the vascular system. Vascular resistance plays a crucial role in regulating blood pressure and blood flow within the body.

Several factors contribute to vascular resistance:

- Vessel Diameter: The diameter of blood vessels is a major determinant of vascular resistance. As vessel diameter decreases, resistance to blood flow increases. This relationship is described by Poiseuille's law, which states that vascular resistance is inversely proportional to the fourth power of vessel radius.

- Vessel Length: Longer blood vessels offer more resistance to blood flow compared to shorter vessels. However, the effect of vessel length on resistance is less significant compared to vessel diameter.

- Blood Viscosity: The thickness or viscosity of blood affects its ability to flow through blood vessels. Higher viscosity leads to increased resistance, as thicker blood encounters more friction against the vessel walls.

- Blood Flow: Increased blood flow through a vessel can lead to increased resistance due to factors such as turbulence or vessel constriction.
- Compliance of Blood Vessels: The compliance, or dispensability, of blood vessels also affects vascular resistance. Stiffer vessels offer greater resistance to blood flow compared to more compliant vessels.

Changes in vascular resistance can have significant physiological implications. For example, increased vascular resistance can lead to hypertension (high blood pressure) and decreased blood flow to organs and tissues. Conversely, decreased vascular resistance can result in hypotension (low blood pressure) and increased blood flow.

Regulation of vascular resistance is complex and involves various mechanisms, including neural, hormonal, and local factors. For instance, the autonomic nervous system regulates vessel diameter through sympathetic and parasympathetic inputs. Hormones such as adrenaline and angiotensin II can also influence vascular tone and resistance. Additionally, local factors such as tissue metabolism and the release of vasoactive substances (e.g., nitric oxide) play a role in regulating vascular resistance in specific tissues and organs.

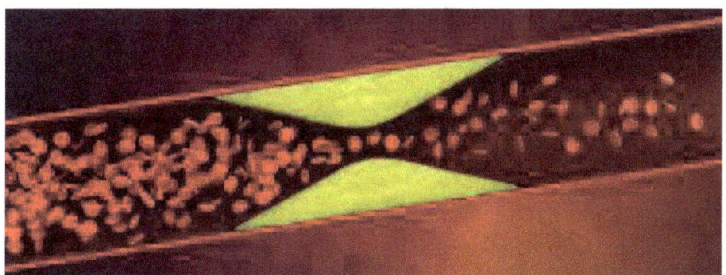

Vascular elasticity refers to the ability of blood vessels to expand and contract in response to changes in blood pressure and blood flow. Elasticity is an essential property of arteries, veins, and other blood vessels, allowing them to accommodate changes in blood volume, maintain adequate blood pressure, and distribute blood throughout the body efficiently.

The elasticity of blood vessels is primarily determined by the composition and structure of their walls, which consist of layers of smooth muscle, elastic fibers, and connective tissue. Key factors that contribute to vascular elasticity *include*:

- Elastic fibers: Blood vessels contain elastic fibers, primarily composed of the protein elastin, which provide resilience and recoil to the vessel walls. These elastic fibers allow arteries to stretch and store potential energy during systole (the contraction phase of the heart cycle) and recoil during diastole (the relaxation phase), helping to maintain continuous blood flow and pressure.

- Smooth muscle tone: Smooth muscle cells in the walls of blood vessels can contract or relax in response to various physiological stimuli, influencing vessel diameter and compliance. Contraction of smooth muscle leads to vasoconstriction, reducing vessel diameter and increasing vascular resistance, while relaxation leads to vasodilation, widening the vessel and reducing resistance.

- Collagen and other extracellular matrix components: Collagen and other structural proteins provide support and stability to blood vessel walls, contributing to their overall strength and elasticity.

Vascular elasticity is crucial for maintaining healthy cardiovascular function. Loss of elasticity, often referred to as arterial stiffness, is a common feature of aging and is associated with various cardiovascular risk factors and diseases, including hypertension, atherosclerosis, and stroke. Arterial stiffness reduces the ability of blood vessels to accommodate changes in blood pressure and flow, leading to increased workload on the heart, impaired tissue perfusion, and elevated cardiovascular risk.

Measures of vascular elasticity, such as pulse wave velocity and arterial compliance, are used clinically to assess arterial stiffness and cardiovascular risk. Lifestyle modifications, such as regular exercise, healthy diet, and avoidance of tobacco use, as well as pharmacological interventions, may help preserve or improve vascular elasticity and reduce cardiovascular risk

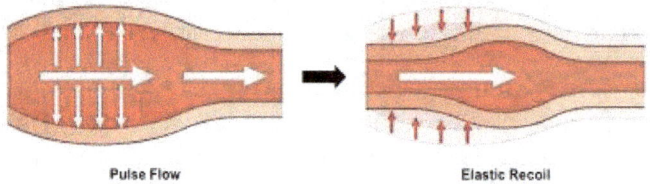

Pulse Flow   Elastic Recoil

Myocardial blood demand refers to the amount of blood flow required by the myocardium, the muscular tissue of the heart, to meet its metabolic needs. The myocardium, like any other tissue in the body, requires a constant supply of oxygen and nutrients to function properly. The demand for blood flow to the myocardium can increase or decrease depending on various factors, *including:*

- Heart rate: An increase in heart rate, such as during exercise or periods of stress, leads to an increased demand for oxygen and nutrients by the myocardium. The heart responds by increasing blood flow to meet this demand.

- Contractility: The forcefulness of myocardial contraction, known as contractility, can also affect myocardial blood demand. Higher contractility requires more oxygen and energy, increasing blood flow to the myocardium.

- Blood pressure: Myocardial blood demand is influenced by systemic blood pressure. Higher blood pressure may increase myocardial oxygen demand, especially during periods of increased cardiac work.

- Cardiac workload: Any condition that increases the workload on the heart, such as hypertension, valvular heart disease, or heart failure, can increase myocardial blood demand.

- Metabolic state: The metabolic state of the myocardium, including factors such as pH, temperature, and concentrations of metabolic substrates, can affect myocardial blood demand. For example, increased metabolic activity during periods of ischemia or hypoxia increases the demand for oxygen and nutrients.

During periods of increased demand, the coronary arteries, which supply blood to the myocardium, dilate to allow for greater blood flow. Coronary blood flow is regulated by various mechanisms, including metabolic factors, neural control, and local vasodilator substances like adenosine and nitric oxide.

Insufficient blood flow to meet myocardial demand can lead to myocardial ischemia, a condition characterized by inadequate oxygen supply to the heart muscle. Prolonged ischemia can result in myocardial infarction (heart attack) and irreversible damage to the myocardium. Therefore, maintaining adequate myocardial blood supply is essential for the normal functioning of the heart.

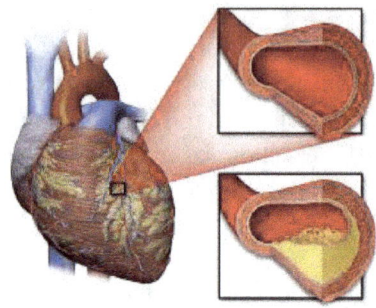

Myocardial blood perfusion volume refers to the volume of blood flow through the coronary arteries to supply the myocardium, the muscular tissue of the heart, with oxygen and nutrients. This perfusion is essential for the normal functioning of the heart, as the myocardium requires a continuous supply of oxygen and nutrients to sustain its metabolic activities.

The coronary arteries are responsible for delivering blood to the myocardium. These arteries branch off from the aorta and encircle the heart, providing oxygenated blood to the heart muscle. During diastole (the relaxation phase of the heart cycle), when the heart is not actively contracting, the coronary arteries fill with blood, allowing for myocardial perfusion.

Several factors influence myocardial blood perfusion volume:

- Coronary artery diameter and patency:
  The diameter of the coronary arteries and their ability to remain open (patent) are crucial determinants of myocardial blood perfusion volume. Narrowing or blockage of coronary arteries due to atherosclerosis or other causes can restrict blood flow to the myocardium, leading to myocardial ischemia and potentially myocardial infarction.

- Coronary blood flow regulation:
  Coronary blood flow is regulated by various factors, including metabolic demand, neural control, and local vasodilator substances like adenosine and nitric oxide. During periods of increased myocardial oxygen demand, such as during exercise or stress, coronary blood flow increases to meet the metabolic needs of the myocardium.

- Blood pressure: Systemic blood pressure influences coronary perfusion pressure, which is the pressure gradient that drives blood flow through the

coronary arteries. Changes in blood pressure can affect myocardial blood perfusion volume.
- Cardiac output: Cardiac output, which is the volume of blood pumped by the heart per unit of time, also affects myocardial blood perfusion volume. An increase in cardiac output typically leads to increased myocardial blood flow to meet the metabolic demands of the heart.

Measurement of myocardial blood perfusion volume is important for assessing cardiac function and diagnosing conditions such as coronary artery disease (CAD) and myocardial ischemia. Techniques such as myocardial perfusion imaging, using modalities like positron emission tomography (PET) or single-photon emission computed tomography (SPECT), can provide information about myocardial blood flow and perfusion abnormalities. Abnormalities in myocardial perfusion volume can indicate areas of reduced blood flow due to coronary artery disease or other cardiac conditions.

Myocardial oxygen consumption (MVO2) refers to the amount of oxygen consumed by the myocardium, the muscular tissue of the heart, to meet its metabolic needs. The heart, like any other muscle in the body, requires oxygen to produce energy (in the form of adenosine triphosphate, or ATP) through aerobic metabolism in order to contract and pump blood throughout the body.

Several factors influence myocardial oxygen consumption:

- Heart rate: Myocardial oxygen consumption is directly proportional to heart rate. An increase in heart rate, such as during exercise or periods of stress, leads to an increased demand for oxygen by the myocardium to support the higher metabolic rate required for increased cardiac output.

- Contractility: The forcefulness of myocardial contraction, known as contractility, also affects myocardial oxygen consumption. Higher contractility requires more energy and oxygen, increasing myocardial oxygen demand.

- Cardiac workload: Myocardial oxygen consumption is influenced by the workload on the heart. Conditions that increase cardiac workload, such as hypertension, valvular heart disease, or heart failure, can increase oxygen demand.

- Afterload: Afterload refers to the resistance against which the heart must pump blood. Increased afterload, such as in hypertension or aortic stenosis, can increase myocardial oxygen consumption.

- Preload: Preload refers to the volume of blood in the heart at the end of diastole, just before the next contraction. Higher preload, such as during fluid overload or in conditions like heart failure, can increase myocardial oxygen consumption.

- Metabolic state: The metabolic state of the myocardium, including factors such as pH, temperature, and concentrations of metabolic substrates, can affect myocardial oxygen consumption. For example, increased metabolic activity during periods of ischemia or hypoxia increases the demand for oxygen and nutrients.

Measurement of myocardial oxygen consumption is important for assessing cardiac function and metabolic demand. It can be estimated indirectly using various techniques, including measurements of oxygen content in arterial and venous blood samples, and calculation of oxygen extraction ratio. Understanding myocardial oxygen consumption is crucial for managing cardiac conditions and optimizing treatment strategies.

Stroke volume (SV) is the amount of blood ejected by the left ventricle of the heart during one contraction, or systole. It represents the difference between the volume of blood in the ventricle at the end of diastole (end-diastolic volume, EDV) and the volume of blood remaining in the ventricle after contraction (end-systolic volume, ESV). Mathematically, stroke volume can be expressed as:

$$SV = EDV - ESV$$

SV is typically measured in milliliters per beat (ml/beat) or in liters per beat (L/beat).

Several factors influence stroke volume:

- Preload: Preload refers to the amount of blood returning to the heart (venous return) and stretching the ventricles during diastole. An increase in preload generally leads to an increase in stroke volume, as the ventricles are filled with a greater volume of blood, allowing for greater ejection during systole. Factors that affect preload include blood volume, venous tone, and ventricular compliance.

- Afterload: Afterload refers to the resistance against which the heart must pump blood during systole. Increased afterload, such as in hypertension or aortic stenosis, can reduce stroke volume by impeding the ejection of blood from the ventricles. Conversely, a decrease in afterload can lead to an increase in stroke volume.

- Contractility: Contractility refers to the forcefulness of myocardial contraction. An increase in contractility leads to a more forceful ejection of blood from the ventricles, resulting in an increase in stroke volume. Factors that influence contractility include sympathetic stimulation, circulating catecholamine (e.g., adrenaline), and medications such as inotropes.

- Heart rate: Heart rate affects stroke volume through its influence on ventricular filling time and diastolic filling. At higher heart rates, there may be less time for ventricular filling, which can decrease stroke volume.

However, the relationship between heart rate and stroke volume is complex and may vary depending on other factors.

Measurement of stroke volume is important for assessing cardiac function and hemodynamic status. It is often measured using various imaging modalities, such as echocardiography or cardiac magnetic resonance imaging (MRI), or calculated using techniques such as the thermo dilution method. Stroke volume is a key determinant of cardiac output, which is the volume of blood pumped by the heart per unit of time, and is essential for maintaining adequate tissue perfusion and oxygen delivery throughout the body.

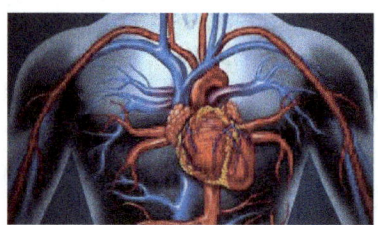

Left ventricular ejection impedance, also known as left ventricular afterload, refers to the resistance that the left ventricle (LV) of the heart must overcome to eject blood into the systemic circulation during systole. Afterload is primarily determined by the pressure in the aorta and the systemic vascular resistance.

Several factors contribute to left ventricular ejection impedance:

- Systemic vascular resistance (SVR): SVR refers to the resistance encountered by blood flow in the systemic circulation. It is influenced by factors such as vessel diameter, vessel length, and blood viscosity. Increased SVR, as seen in conditions like hypertension or vasoconstriction, increases afterload and makes it more difficult for the left ventricle to eject blood into the aorta.

- Aortic pressure: Aortic pressure represents the pressure against which the left ventricle must pump blood during systole. Higher aortic pressure, as seen in conditions like hypertension or aortic stenosis, increases left ventricular afterload.

- Aortic compliance: Aortic compliance refers to the ability of the aorta to expand and recoil in response to changes in blood volume. Reduced aortic compliance, as seen in aging or atherosclerosis, can increase left ventricular afterload by increasing impedance to left ventricular ejection.

Left ventricular ejection impedance plays a crucial role in determining stroke volume and cardiac output. The left ventricle must generate sufficient force to overcome afterload in order to effectively eject blood into the systemic circulation. High afterload can lead to increased myocardial oxygen consumption, left ventricular hypertrophy, and impaired cardiac function over time.

Measurement of left ventricular ejection impedance can be challenging and is often estimated indirectly. Indices such as systemic vascular resistance (SVR), arterial pressure, and ventricular pressure-volume loops can provide information about afterload and its impact on left ventricular function. Management of conditions that increase afterload, such as hypertension or aortic stenosis, may involve medications or interventions aimed at reducing vascular resistance or lowering aortic pressure to improve cardiac function and outcomes.

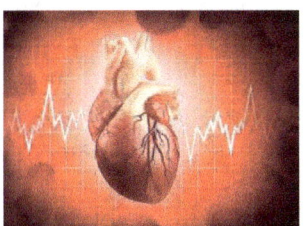

Left ventricular effective pump power refers to the ability of the left ventricle (LV) of the heart to generate mechanical work during systole to pump blood into the systemic circulation. It is a measure of the energy output of the left ventricle and reflects its contractile function and efficiency in ejecting blood.

The calculation of left ventricular effective pump power involves several variables, including stroke volume (SV), mean arterial pressure (MAP), heart rate (HR), and the efficiency of the left ventricle in converting mechanical energy into work. The formula for calculating left ventricular effective pump power is:

$$P = HR \times SV \times MAP \times 451$$

Where:

P represents left ventricular effective pump power in watts (W).

SV represents stroke volume, the amount of blood ejected by the left ventricle per beat, typically measured in milliliters (mL).

MAP represents mean arterial pressure, the average pressure in the systemic arteries during one cardiac cycle, typically measured in millimeters of mercury (mmHg).

HR represents heart rate, the number of heart beats per minute.

The constant 451 is a conversion factor used to convert units to watts.

Left ventricular effective pump power provides insight into the mechanical performance of the left ventricle and its ability to meet the demands of the body's circulation. Changes in left ventricular effective pump power can occur in various cardiovascular conditions, such as heart failure, myocardial infarction, or valvular heart disease, and can impact overall cardiac function and patient outcomes.

Assessment of left ventricular effective pump power can aid in the diagnosis, management, and prognosis of cardiovascular diseases. It is often evaluated alongside other measures of cardiac function, such as ejection fraction, cardiac output, and hemodynamic parameters, to provide a comprehensive assessment of heart function.

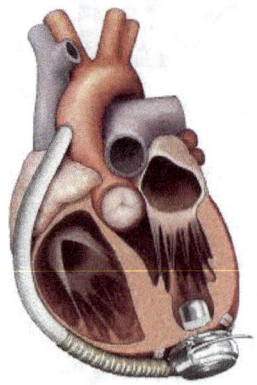

Coronary artery elasticity refers to the ability of the coronary arteries to stretch and recoil in response to changes in blood flow and pressure. Elasticity is an essential property of arteries, including the coronary arteries, as it allows them to accommodate changes in blood volume, maintain adequate blood flow, and distribute blood to the heart muscle efficiently.

The elasticity of coronary arteries is primarily determined by the composition and structure of their walls, which consist of layers of smooth muscle, elastic fibers, and connective tissue. *Key factors that contribute to coronary artery elasticity include:*

- Elastic fibers: Coronary arteries contain elastic fibers, primarily composed of the protein elastin, which provide resilience and recoil to the artery walls. These elastic fibers allow coronary arteries to stretch during systole (when the heart contracts) and recoil during diastole (when the heart relaxes), helping to maintain continuous blood flow and pressure to the heart muscle.

- Smooth muscle tone: Smooth muscle cells in the walls of coronary arteries can contract or relax in response to various physiological stimuli, influencing artery diameter and compliance. Contraction of smooth muscle leads to vasoconstriction, reducing artery diameter and increasing vascular resistance, while relaxation leads to vasodilation, widening the artery and reducing resistance.

- Endothelial function: The endothelium, the innermost layer of the coronary artery wall, plays a crucial role in regulating vascular tone and elasticity. Endothelial cells release vasodilator substances such as nitric oxide, which promote relaxation of smooth muscle cells and enhance artery elasticity.

- Collagen and other extracellular matrix components: Collagen and other structural proteins provide support and stability to coronary artery walls, contributing to their overall strength and elasticity.

Maintaining optimal coronary artery elasticity is important for ensuring adequate blood flow and oxygen delivery to the heart muscle, especially during periods of increased demand such as exercise or stress. Reduced coronary artery elasticity, often associated with aging, atherosclerosis, or other cardiovascular risk factors, can lead to impaired coronary blood flow, increased myocardial oxygen demand, and an elevated risk of cardiovascular events such as myocardial infarction or angina.

Assessment of coronary artery elasticity is challenging and often inferred indirectly from measures such as pulse wave velocity, arterial compliance, or coronary flow reserve. Lifestyle modifications, medications, and interventions aimed at preserving or improving coronary artery elasticity may help reduce cardiovascular risk and improve overall heart health.

GASTROINTESTINAL FUNCTION

Pepsin is a digestive enzyme produced by the chief cells in the stomach's gastric glands. It plays a crucial role in breaking down proteins into smaller peptides, which can then be further digested into amino acids by other enzymes in the digestive tract.

The secretion of pepsin is regulated by several factors, including:

- Gastric Acid: Pepsinogen, the inactive precursor of pepsin, is released into the stomach lumen by chief cells. Upon exposure to the acidic environment of the stomach, particularly hydrochloric acid (HCl), pepsinogen is converted into active pepsin.

- Gastric Hormones: Hormones such as gastrin, produced by specialized cells in the stomach and small intestine, stimulate the secretion of gastric acid and pepsinogen by the gastric glands.

- Neural Regulation: Neural signals from the vagus nerve, as well as local enteric nervous system reflexes, can influence the secretion of gastric juices, including pepsinogen.
- Presence of Proteins: The presence of proteins in the stomach stimulates the release of gastrin, which in turn enhances the secretion of pepsinogen and gastric acid.

While there isn't a specific "pepsin secretion coefficient" in standard biological terminology, researchers and clinicians may use various measures and assays to assess pepsin activity or secretion levels in the context of digestive function or gastrointestinal disorders. These may include techniques such as enzyme assays, immunohistochemistry, or molecular biology methods to quantify pepsin expression or activity.

The function of gastric peristalsis, which is the coordinated, rhythmic contraction and relaxation of muscles in the stomach wall that helps to mix and propel food along the digestive tract.

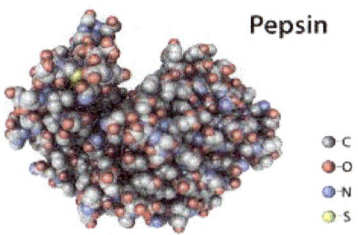

Gastric peristalsis serves several important functions in digestion:

- Mixing: The contractions of the stomach muscles help to mix ingested food with gastric juices, including hydrochloric acid and digestive enzymes, facilitating the breakdown of food particles and aiding in digestion.

- Grinding: Peristaltic contractions help to mechanically break down food into smaller particles, increasing its surface area and exposing it to digestive enzymes for more efficient digestion.

- Emptying: Gastric peristalsis propels partially digested food from the stomach into the small intestine, allowing for further digestion and absorption of nutrients. This process is known as gastric emptying.

Several factors can influence the function of gastric peristalsis:

- Neural Regulation: The enteric nervous system, which is a complex network of neurons within the gastrointestinal tract, coordinates gastric motility, including peristalsis. Neural signals from the brain, as well as local reflex arcs, regulate the timing and intensity of gastric contractions.

- Hormonal Regulation: Gastric peristalsis is also influenced by hormonal signals, such as gastrin, released in response to the presence of food in the stomach. Gastrin stimulates gastric acid secretion and enhances gastric motility to aid in digestion.

- Stretch Reflex: The stretching of the stomach wall due to food intake triggers reflexive contractions known as the "gastric stretch reflex," which promotes gastric peristalsis and gastric emptying.

- Composition of Food: The type and composition of ingested food can affect the rate and pattern of gastric peristalsis. For example, foods high in fat or protein may delay gastric emptying compared to carbohydrates.
- Psychological Factors: Emotional states, stress, and anxiety can influence gastric motility through neural pathways, leading to changes in peristaltic activity.

While there isn't a single coefficient that quantifies gastric peristalsis function, clinicians and researchers may use various methods to assess gastric motility and function, including imaging studies, manometer, and scintigraphy, to evaluate peristaltic activity and gastric emptying rates in clinical settings

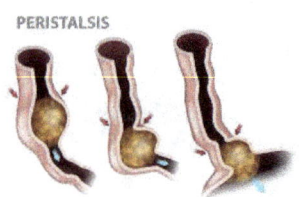

Gastric absorption refers to the process by which nutrients, water, electrolytes, and other substances are absorbed from the stomach into the bloodstream. While the stomach is primarily responsible for the digestion of food, it also plays a role in the absorption of certain substances, although the majority of absorption occurs in the small intestine.

Factors that influence gastric absorption include:

- Surface Area: The surface area available for absorption in the stomach lining is relatively small compared to the extensive surface area of the small intestine, which is specialized for absorption. Therefore, the stomach's contribution to overall absorption is limited.

- Permeability: The stomach lining is less permeable than the lining of the small intestine. While some substances, such as water, electrolytes, and certain drugs (like alcohol and aspirin), can be absorbed in the stomach to some extent, the absorption of nutrients like carbohydrates, proteins, and fats primarily occurs in the small intestine.

- Gastric Emptying Rate: The rate at which the stomach empties its contents into the small intestine can affect absorption. Rapid gastric emptying may reduce the time available for absorption in the stomach, while delayed emptying can prolong exposure to ingested substances and potentially enhance absorption.

- pH Environment: The stomach's acidic environment, maintained by gastric acid (hydrochloric acid), can influence the solubility and absorption of certain substances. Some substances may be better absorbed in an acidic environment, while others may require a more neutral pH for optimal absorption.

- Presence of Food: The presence of food in the stomach can affect gastric absorption. For example, the presence of carbohydrates can stimulate the

release of hormones like gastrin and insulin, which may influence gastric motility and absorption processes.
- Chemical Properties of Substances: The chemical properties of ingested substances, such as their molecular size, polarity, and solubility, can influence their absorption characteristics in the stomach.

While the stomach does contribute to the absorption of some substances, its primary function is digestion rather than absorption. Most absorption occurs in the small intestine, where the intestinal lining is highly specialized for nutrient absorption through processes like passive diffusion, facilitated diffusion, active transport, and endocytosis.

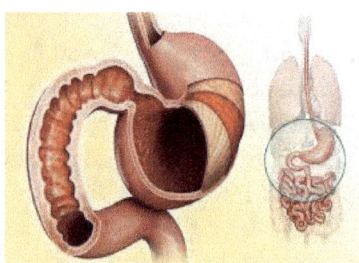

Peristalsis in the small intestine refers to the coordinated muscular contractions and relaxations that propel chime (partially digested food mixed with gastric juices) through the small intestine for further digestion and absorption of nutrients. This process is essential for the movement of nutrients along the digestive tract and eventual elimination of waste.

Factors that influence small intestine peristalsis include:

- Neural Regulation: The enteric nervous system, which is a complex network of neurons within the gastrointestinal tract, coordinates peristalsis in the small intestine. Neural signals from the brain, as well as local reflex arcs, regulate the timing and intensity of peristaltic contractions.

- Hormonal Regulation: Hormones such as motile, released by specialized cells in the small intestine, stimulate peristalsis and help regulate gastrointestinal motility. Other hormones, including serotonin and cholecystokinin (CCK), may also influence intestinal motility indirectly.

- Stretch Reflex: The stretching of the intestinal wall due to the presence of chime triggers reflexive contractions known as the "intestinal stretch reflex," which promotes peristalsis and propels chime along the small intestine.

- Gastrointestinal Hormones: Hormones released in response to the presence of nutrients in the small intestine, such as gastrin and secretin, can affect intestinal motility and secretion, facilitating digestion and absorption.

- Composition of Chime: The type and composition of chime entering the small intestine can influence peristalsis. For example, the presence of fats or proteins may trigger the release of specific hormones that modulate intestinal motility and digestive enzyme secretion.

- Microbial Factors: The gut micro biota, which consists of trillions of bacteria residing in the intestines, can also influence intestinal motility through their metabolic activities and interactions with the host's immune system.

- Psychological Factors: Emotional states, stress, and anxiety can influence gastrointestinal motility through neural pathways, leading to changes in peristaltic activity in the small intestine.

While there isn't a single coefficient that quantifies small intestine peristalsis function, clinicians and researchers may use various methods to assess intestinal motility and function, including imaging studies, manometer, and transit time tests, to evaluate peristaltic activity and transit rates in clinical settings.

The small intestine is the primary site for the absorption of nutrients, water, electrolytes, and other substances from digested food. This absorption occurs across the specialized epithelial lining of the small intestine, which is characterized by numerous finger-like projections called villi and even smaller microvilli on the surface of absorptive cells. These structures significantly increase the surface area available for absorption.

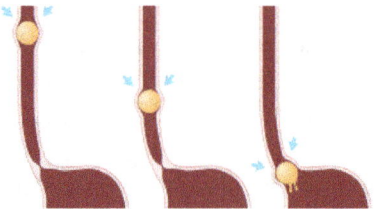

Factors that influence small intestine absorption include:

- Surface Area: The extensive surface area provided by the villi and microvilli allows for efficient absorption of nutrients. This large surface area maximizes contact between digested food and the absorptive cells lining the small intestine.

- Transport Mechanisms: Various transport mechanisms facilitate the absorption of different nutrients across the epithelial cells of the small intestine. These mechanisms include passive diffusion, facilitated diffusion, active transport, and secondary active transport (cotransport).

- Nutrient Concentration: The concentration gradient of nutrients between the intestinal lumen and the bloodstream affects the rate and efficiency of absorption. Higher concentrations of nutrients in the intestinal lumen can promote faster absorption.

- Digestive Enzymes: Digestive enzymes released by the pancreas and brush border enzymes produced by the small intestine help break down complex nutrients into smaller, absorbable molecules. Optimal enzyme activity is crucial for efficient absorption.

- pH Environment: The pH environment of the small intestine, which is regulated by pancreatic secretions and bile, can affect the solubility and absorption of certain nutrients. Some nutrients may be better absorbed under acidic conditions, while others may require a more alkaline environment.

- Intestinal Motility: Peristaltic contractions of the small intestine help mix the contents and bring them into contact with the absorptive surface. Proper intestinal motility ensures adequate exposure of digested food to absorptive cells.

- Intestinal Transit Time: The rate at which digested food moves through the small intestine, known as intestinal transit time, can influence absorption. Prolonged transit time may lead to increased absorption of water and electrolytes but could decrease nutrient absorption if the chime spends insufficient time in contact with the absorptive surface.

- Intestinal Permeability: The permeability of the intestinal epithelium can affect the absorption of nutrients. Disruption of the intestinal barrier, as seen in conditions like inflammatory bowel disease or celiac disease, can impair nutrient absorption.

While there isn't a single coefficient to quantify small intestine absorption function, clinicians and researchers may use various methods to assess intestinal absorption, such as absorption tests, fecal analysis, and serum nutrient levels, to evaluate nutrient absorption efficiency in clinical settings

LARGE INTESTINE FUNCTION

Peristalsis in the large intestine, also known as colonic motility, refers to the rhythmic contractions and relaxations of the muscles in the colon that propel fecal matter through the digestive tract toward the rectum for elimination. This process helps to mix the contents of the colon, absorb water, and consolidate waste material.

Factors that influence large intestine peristalsis include:

- Neural Regulation: The enteric nervous system, which is a complex network of neurons within the gastrointestinal tract, coordinates colonic motility. Neural signals from the brain, as well as local reflex arcs, regulate the timing and intensity of peristaltic contractions.

- Hormonal Regulation: Hormones such as serotonin and motile, released by specialized cells in the gastrointestinal tract, help regulate colonic motility. For example, motile stimulates colonic contractions during fasting periods to clear the intestines.

- Stretch Reflex: The stretching of the colon wall due to the presence of fecal matter triggers reflexive contractions known as the "gastro colic reflex," which promotes peristalsis and moves fecal material through the colon.

- Dietary Factors: The composition and volume of ingested food can affect colonic motility. High-fiber foods, for example, can stimulate peristalsis and promote regular bowel movements, while low-fiber diets may lead to slower transit times and constipation.

- Hydration Status: Adequate hydration is important for maintaining normal colonic motility and preventing constipation. Dehydration can lead to harder stools and slower transit times through the colon.

- Physical Activity: Regular physical activity can help promote healthy colonic motility by stimulating bowel movements and reducing the risk of constipation.

- Medications: Certain medications, such as laxatives, antidiarrheal, and opioids, can affect colonic motility and bowel function. For example, opioids can slow down peristalsis and lead to constipation.

- Gut Micro biota: The gut micro biota, which consists of trillions of bacteria residing in the colon, can influence colonic motility through their metabolic activities and interactions with the host's immune system.

While there isn't a specific coefficient that quantifies large intestine peristalsis function, clinicians and researchers may use various methods to assess colonic motility, such as colon transit studies, manometer, and imaging techniques, to evaluate peristaltic activity and transit rates in clinical settings

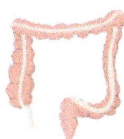

The colon, or large intestine, primarily functions in the reabsorption of water and electrolytes from undigested food material (feces) to form solid waste for elimination. While the primary role of the colon is water absorption, it also absorbs small amounts of other substances, such as short-chain fatty acids and electrolytes.

Factors that influence colonic absorption include:

- Water and Electrolyte Balance: The primary function of the colon is to reabsorb water and electrolytes from the remaining digestive material. This process is crucial for maintaining fluid and electrolyte balance in the body.

- Microbial Fermentation: The colon is home to trillions of bacteria, collectively known as the gut micro biota, which play a significant role in fermenting undigested carbohydrates and fiber. This fermentation process produces short-chain fatty acids (SCFAs), such as acetate, propionate, and butyrate, which can be absorbed and used as an energy source by the colonocytes (cells lining the colon).

- Ion Transporters: Transport proteins located on the surface of colonocytes facilitate the absorption of electrolytes such as sodium, chloride, potassium, and bicarbonate. These ion transporters help maintain electrolyte balance and regulate fluid absorption in the colon.

- Dietary Fiber: Fiber-rich foods, such as fruits, vegetables, and whole grains, can affect colonic absorption by increasing fecal bulk, promoting regular bowel movements, and providing substrate for microbial fermentation. Some soluble fibers can also bind to water and form a gel-like substance, which may enhance water retention in the colon.

- Hydration Status: Adequate hydration is essential for maintaining normal colonic function and absorption. Dehydration can lead to harder stools and slower transit times through the colon, potentially affecting absorption efficiency.

- Colonic Transit Time: The rate at which fecal material moves through the colon, known as colonic transit time, can influence absorption. Prolonged transit times may lead to increased water reabsorption and firmer stools, while rapid transit times may result in decreased absorption and looser stools.

- Gastrointestinal Motility: Colonic motility, including peristaltic contractions and mass movements, can affect absorption by promoting mixing and contact between fecal material and the colonic mucosa.

While there isn't a specific coefficient that quantifies colonic absorption, researchers and clinicians may use various methods to assess colonic function and absorption efficiency, such as fecal water content analysis, colonic transit studies, and measurement of electrolyte concentrations in fecal samples. These assessments can provide valuable insights into colonic health and function.

The gut micro biota refers to the diverse community of microorganisms, including bacteria, archaic, viruses, and fungi, that reside in the gastrointestinal tract, primarily in the large intestine (colon). These microorganisms play essential roles in digestion, metabolism, immune function, and overall health.

Factors that influence the composition and function of the gut micro biota include:

- Diet: Diet is one of the most significant determinants of gut micro biota composition. Different dietary components, such as fiber, carbohydrates, fats, and protein, can selectively enrich certain bacterial species while inhibiting others. A diverse diet rich in fiber and plant-based foods tends to promote a more diverse and beneficial gut micro biota.

- Antibiotic Use: Antibiotics can disrupt the balance of the gut micro biota by killing beneficial bacteria along with pathogenic ones. This can lead to dysbiosis, an imbalance in the gut micro biota associated with various health problems. The effects of antibiotics on the gut micro biota can be long-lasting, and in some cases, may persist even after antibiotic treatment has ended.

- Host Genetics: Host genetics play a role in shaping the composition of the gut micro biota. Certain genetic factors influence susceptibility to colonization by specific bacterial species and may affect interactions between the host and its micro biota.

- Age: The composition of the gut micro biota undergoes significant changes throughout life, from infancy to old age. Early-life factors, such as mode of delivery (vaginal birth vs. cesarean section) and feeding practices (breastfeeding vs. formula feeding), can have long-lasting effects on the development of the gut micro biota.

- Environmental Exposures: Environmental factors, including exposure to pollutants, toxins, and dietary additives, can influence the composition and function of the gut micro biota. Additionally, lifestyle factors such as stress, physical activity, and sleep patterns may also impact the gut micro biota.

- Medications and Medical Interventions: Certain medications, such as proton pump inhibitors, no steroidal anti-inflammatory drugs (NSAIDs), and chemotherapy agents, can alter the gut micro biota. Medical interventions, such as surgery, radiation therapy, and fecal micro biota transplantation, can also have profound effects on gut micro biota composition and function.

- Immune System: The host immune system plays a crucial role in shaping the gut micro biota and maintaining its homeostasis. Interactions between the immune system and the gut micro biota are bidirectional, with the micro biota influencing immune development and function, and the immune system modulating the composition and activity of the micro biota.

While there isn't a specific coefficient that quantifies the gut micro biota, researchers use various techniques, such as DNA sequencing, met genomics, and metabolomics, to study the composition, diversity, and function of the gut micro biota in health and disease. These studies have provided valuable insights into the role of the gut micro biota in human health and have led to the development of new therapeutic approaches targeting the micro biota.

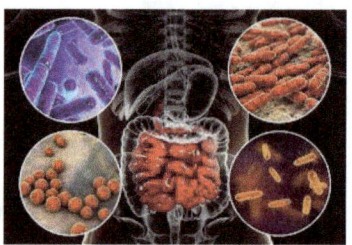

Intraluminal pressure refers to the pressure within the lumen or cavity of a hollow organ or structure, such as the gastrointestinal tract or blood vessels. This pressure can vary depending on factors such as the state of contraction or relaxation of the surrounding muscles, the presence of contents within the lumen, and any obstructions or abnormalities affecting the organ.

For example, in the gastrointestinal tract, intraluminal pressure can fluctuate as a result of peristaltic contractions, which propel food and digestive juices through the digestive system. Additionally, the presence of gas, fluid, or fecal material within the intestines can affect intraluminal pressure.

Factors that may influence intraluminal pressure in the gastrointestinal tract include:

- Peristalsis: Rhythmic contractions of the smooth muscle in the walls of the gastrointestinal tract generate waves of pressure that move material along the digestive tract. Stronger contractions can increase intraluminal pressure and facilitate the movement of contents through the intestines.

- Presence of Contents: The presence of food, fluids, gas, or fecal material within the intestines can affect intraluminal pressure. For example, a buildup of gas or feces can increase pressure and contribute to symptoms such as bloating or discomfort.

- Obstructions: Blockages or obstructions within the gastrointestinal tract, such as tumors, strictures, or impacted feces, can disrupt normal peristalsis and cause changes in intraluminal pressure. This can lead to symptoms such as abdominal pain, distension, or vomiting.

- Functional Disorders: Conditions affecting gastrointestinal motility, such as irritable bowel syndrome (IBS) or gastroparesis, can alter intraluminal pressure and contribute to symptoms such as abdominal pain, bloating, and changes in bowel habits.

- Neurological Disorders: Damage or dysfunction of the nerves that control gastrointestinal motility, such as in conditions like Parkinson's disease or diabetic neuropathy, can affect intraluminal pressure and disrupt normal digestive function.

- Medications: Certain medications, such as antispasmodics or laxatives, can affect gastrointestinal motility and intraluminal pressure. For example, laxatives may increase intraluminal pressure to promote bowel movements, while antispasmodics may reduce pressure and relieve symptoms of abdominal cramping.

While the term "intraluminal pressure coefficient" may not be commonly used, clinicians and researchers may use various methods to measure and assess intraluminal pressure in the gastrointestinal tract, such as manometer, imaging studies, or direct pressure measurements during endoscopy or surgery. These assessments can provide valuable information for diagnosing and managing gastrointestinal disorders.

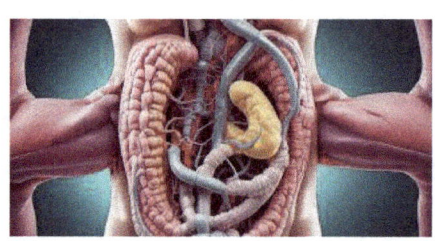

LIVER FUNCTION

Protein metabolism refers to the biochemical processes involved in the synthesis, breakdown, and utilization of proteins in the body. Proteins are macromolecules composed of amino acids, and they play essential roles in numerous biological functions, including structural support, enzymatic activity, immune function, and cell signaling.

Protein metabolism consists of two main processes: protein synthesis (anabolism) and protein breakdown (catabolism). These processes are tightly regulated to maintain protein homeostasis in the body.

Protein Synthesis (Anabolism):

Protein synthesis involves the formation of new proteins from individual amino acids, which are linked together in a specific sequence dictated by the genetic code.

The process of protein synthesis occurs primarily in ribosomes, cellular structures where mRNA (messenger RNA) serves as a template for protein production.

Protein synthesis is an energy-intensive process that requires ATP (adenosine triphosphate) as an energy source, as well as specific enzymes and molecular chaperones to facilitate protein folding and assembly.

The rate of protein synthesis is influenced by various factors, including dietary protein intake, hormonal signaling (e.g., insulin, growth hormone), cellular signaling pathways (e.g., motor pathway), and physiological state (e.g., growth, recovery from injury).

Protein Breakdown (Catabolism):

Protein breakdown involves the degradation of proteins into their constituent amino acids or smaller peptide fragments.

The primary mechanism of protein breakdown is proteolysis, which is carried out by enzymes called proteases. Proteases cleave peptide bonds between amino acids, resulting in the release of amino acids.

Protein breakdown occurs continuously in the body as part of normal cellular turnover and protein recycling. Additionally, during periods of nutrient deprivation or metabolic stress (e.g., fasting, exercise, illness), protein breakdown may increase to provide amino acids for energy production or gluconeogenesis (the synthesis of glucose from non-carbohydrate sources).

The rate of protein breakdown is regulated by various factors, including hormonal signaling (e.g., cortisol, glucagon), cellular energy status (e.g., ATP levels), and nutrient availability (e.g., amino acid availability, dietary protein intake).

Protein Utilization and Turnover:

Once amino acids are released through protein breakdown, they can be utilized for various purposes, including energy production, synthesis of new proteins, or conversion into other biomolecules (e.g., glucose, fatty acids).

The balance between protein synthesis and breakdown determines protein turnover, which refers to the rate at which proteins are synthesized and degraded within the body.

Protein turnover is essential for maintaining cellular function, tissue repair, and adaptation to changing physiological demands. Imbalances in protein turnover can lead to alterations in body composition, muscle wasting (cachexia), or impaired tissue repair.

Overall, protein metabolism is a dynamic and tightly regulated process essential for maintaining cellular function, tissue homeostasis, and overall health. Proper nutrition, including an adequate intake of dietary protein and essential amino acids, is crucial for supporting protein synthesis and turnover, particularly during periods of growth, development, and recovery from injury or illness.

Energy production refers to the process by which cells convert various forms of energy-containing molecules into adenosine triphosphate (ATP), the universal currency of cellular energy. ATP is utilized by cells to perform various physiological functions, including muscle contraction, active transport, biosynthesis, and cell signaling. The process of energy production occurs primarily through cellular respiration, which involves the breakdown of nutrients such as carbohydrates, fats, and proteins to generate ATP.

Here's an overview of the main pathways involved in energy production:

Glycolysis:

Glycolysis is the initial stage of cellular respiration that takes place in the cytoplasm of cells.

In glycolysis, glucose (a six-carbon sugar) is broken down into two molecules of pyruvate (a three-carbon compound).

During this process, a small amount of ATP is generated, and NADH (reduced nicotinamide adenine dinucleotide) is produced as a coenzyme.

Glycolysis can occur under aerobic (with oxygen) or anaerobic (without oxygen) conditions, depending on the availability of oxygen.

Pyruvate Oxidation:

In aerobic conditions, pyruvate produced during glycolysis enters the mitochondria, where it undergoes further oxidation.

Pyruvate is converted into acetyl-CoA (acetyl coenzyme A) by a multienzyme complex called the pyruvate dehydrogenase complex.

This step generates NADH and releases carbon dioxide as a byproduct.

Citric Acid Cycle (Krebs cycle):

Acetyl-CoA enters the citric acid cycle, a series of enzymatic reactions that occur within the mitochondrial matrix.

During the citric acid cycle, acetyl-CoA is oxidized to produce carbon dioxide, generating NADH and FADH2 (reduced flavin adenine dinucleotide) as electron carriers.

The citric acid cycle also produces a small amount of ATP through substrate-level phosphorylation.

Electron Transport Chain (ETC):

The electrons carried by NADH and FADH2 are transferred to the electron transport chain, located in the inner mitochondrial membrane.

As electrons move through the electron transport chain, they release energy, which is used to pump protons (H+) across the inner mitochondrial membrane, creating an electrochemical gradient.

The flow of protons back across the membrane through ATP synthase drives the synthesis of ATP from ADP (adenosine triphosphate) and inorganic phosphate in a process known as oxidative phosphorylation.

Oxygen serves as the final electron acceptor in the electron transport chain, combining with electrons and protons to form water.

Overall, cellular respiration is the primary pathway for energy production in cells, generating ATP through the oxidation of nutrients. In addition to glucose, fats and proteins can also be utilized as energy sources through various metabolic pathways that feed into the citric acid cycle and electron transport chain. The efficient functioning of these metabolic pathways is essential for maintaining cellular energy homeostasis and supporting physiological processes throughout the body.

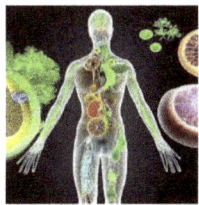

Detoxification is a complex physiological process by which the body eliminates or neutralizes harmful substances, including toxins, drugs, pollutants, and metabolic waste products. It involves multiple organs, tissues, and biochemical pathways working together to identify, transform, and eliminate harmful substances from the body.

Key organs involved in detoxification include:

- Liver: The liver is the primary organ responsible for detoxification. It performs a wide range of metabolic functions, including the synthesis of enzymes and proteins involved in detoxification pathways. The liver detoxifies harmful substances through two main phases: Phase I and Phase II metabolism.

- Phase I Metabolism (Functionalization): In this phase, enzymes such as cytochrome P450 (CYP450) enzymes oxidize, reduce, or hydrolyze toxic compounds to make them more water-soluble and easier to excrete. This process can generate reactive intermediates, which may be further metabolized in Phase II.

- Phase II Metabolism (Conjugation): Conjugation reactions involve the attachment of water-soluble molecules (e.g., glucuronic acid, sulfate, glutathione) to Phase I metabolites, forming conjugates that are more readily excreted in bile or urine.

- Kidneys: The kidneys filter blood and eliminate waste products, excess electrolytes, and water from the body through urine. They play a crucial role in excreting water-soluble metabolites produced during detoxification, particularly those formed in Phase II metabolism in the liver.

- Intestines: The intestines are involved in the elimination of toxins and waste products through feces. Bile, produced by the liver and stored in the gallbladder, contains conjugated toxins and is released into the intestines to aid in the digestion and elimination of fat-soluble compounds.

- Skin: The skin serves as a barrier to environmental toxins and can eliminate certain waste products through sweat. Sweating during physical activity or in a sauna can promote the excretion of water-soluble toxins through the skin.

- Lungs: The lungs eliminate volatile compounds and gases from the body through exhalation. While the lungs are not primarily involved in detoxification, they play a role in eliminating volatile toxins absorbed through inhalation.

Detoxification pathways can be influenced by various factors, including genetics, diet, lifestyle, environmental exposures, and overall health status. Certain nutrients and phytochemicals found in fruits, vegetables, and herbs may support detoxification processes by providing essential cofactors and antioxidants.

It's important to note that while the body has natural detoxification mechanisms, there is limited scientific evidence supporting the efficacy of many commercial detox products or extreme detox diets. Maintaining a balanced diet, staying hydrated, engaging in regular physical activity, minimizing exposure to toxins, and avoiding excessive alcohol and drug use are important strategies for supporting overall health and optimizing natural detoxification processes. Individuals with specific health concerns or exposure to toxins should consult with healthcare professionals for personalized guidance on detoxification and health maintenance.

- Bile secretion is a critical physiological process carried out by the liver to produce and release bile into the digestive system. Bile is a complex fluid composed of water, bile salts, bile pigments, cholesterol, phospholipids, and electrolytes. It plays several essential roles in digestion, nutrient absorption, and waste excretion. Here's an overview of bile secretion and its functions:

- Liver Production: Bile is primarily produced by hepatocytes, the liver cells. Hepatocytes synthesize bile salts, cholesterol, and phospholipids, which are the primary components of bile. Bile salts, particularly bile acids (formed from cholesterol), are critical for emulsifying dietary fats and aiding in their digestion and absorption.

- Bile Ducts: Bile produced by hepatocytes is secreted into small bile ducts within the liver. These bile ducts merge to form larger bile ducts, eventually leading to the common bile duct, which transports bile out of the liver and into the small intestine.

- Gallbladder Storage: Bile produced by the liver can either flow directly into the common bile duct or be diverted into the gallbladder for storage and concentration. In the gallbladder, bile is concentrated by reabsorbing water and electrolytes, making it more potent for digestion.

- Bile Release: When needed for digestion, bile is released from the gallbladder into the duodenum (the first part of the small intestine) in response to hormonal and neural signals triggered by the presence of food, particularly fatty food. The hormone cholecystokinin (CCK), released by the duodenum in response to fat and protein intake, stimulates the contraction of the gallbladder and relaxation of the sphincter of Oddi (the muscular valve controlling bile release into the small intestine).

- Digestion and Absorption: Bile plays a crucial role in the digestion and absorption of dietary fats and fat-soluble vitamins (A, D, E, and K). Bile salts emulsify large fat droplets into smaller micelles, increasing the surface area for the action of pancreatic lipase, an enzyme that breaks down triglycerides into fatty acids and monoglycerides. This process enhances the absorption of fatty acids and fat-soluble vitamins by the intestinal mucosa.

- Waste Excretion: Bile also serves as a route for excreting waste products, including bilirubin, a breakdown product of heme (from hemoglobin and other heme-containing proteins). Bilirubin gives bile its characteristic yellow-green color. Excess bilirubin can lead to jaundice, a yellowing of the skin and eyes.

Overall, bile secretion is essential for the digestion and absorption of fats and fat-soluble vitamins, as well as for the elimination of waste products from the body. Dysfunction in bile secretion can lead to digestive disorders, impaired nutrient absorption, and other health problems.

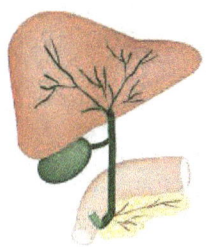

Liver fat content refers to the amount of fat stored in the liver tissue. Normally, the liver contains some fat, but when the amount of fat stored exceeds a certain threshold, it can lead to a condition known as hepatic steatosis or fatty liver disease. *There are two main types of fatty liver disease:*

- Non-alcoholic Fatty Liver Disease (NAFLD): This is the most common form of liver disease in which excessive fat accumulates in the liver of people who drink little to no alcohol. NAFLD encompasses a spectrum of liver conditions, ranging from simple fatty liver (steatosis) to non-alcoholic steatohepatitis (NASH), which involves inflammation and liver cell damage. NAFLD is closely associated with obesity, insulin resistance, metabolic syndrome, and type 2 diabetes.

- Alcoholic Fatty Liver Disease (AFLD): This condition occurs due to excessive alcohol consumption, leading to fat accumulation in the liver. Similar to NAFLD, AFLD can progress from simple fatty liver to more severe forms of liver damage, including alcoholic hepatitis and cirrhosis. The risk and severity of AFLD depend on factors such as the amount and duration of alcohol consumption, genetics, and other concurrent liver diseases.

The measurement of liver fat content can be assessed through various methods, including imaging techniques and blood tests. *Common methods for assessing liver fat include:*

- Imaging Techniques: Imaging modalities such as ultrasound, computed tomography (CT), and magnetic resonance imaging (MRI) can provide non-invasive assessments of liver fat content. MRI techniques like magnetic resonance spectroscopy (MRS) and magnetic resonance imaging-estimated proton density fat fraction (MRI-PDFF) are particularly accurate for quantifying liver fat.

- Blood Tests: Blood tests may measure biomarkers associated with liver fat accumulation, such as alanine aminotransferase (ALT) and aspartate aminotransferase (AST) levels. Elevated levels of these enzymes may indicate liver inflammation or damage, which can be associated with fatty liver disease.

- Liver Biopsy: Liver biopsy involves the removal of a small sample of liver tissue for microscopic examination. It is considered the gold standard for diagnosing and staging liver diseases, including fatty liver disease. However, liver biopsy is an invasive procedure and may not be suitable for routine monitoring of liver fat content.

Monitoring and managing liver fat content is essential for preventing the progression of fatty liver disease and reducing the risk of complications such as liver fibrosis, cirrhosis, and liver cancer. Lifestyle modifications, including weight loss, dietary changes, regular exercise, and limiting alcohol consumption, are often recommended as first-line treatments for fatty liver disease. In some cases, medications or surgical interventions may be necessary to manage underlying metabolic conditions or complications of advanced liver disease. Individuals with concerns about liver health should consult with healthcare professionals for appropriate evaluation and management.

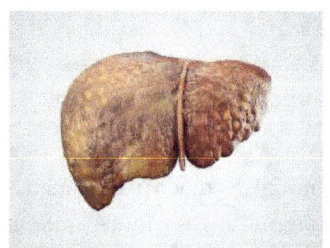

GALLBLADDER FUNCTION

Serum globulin refers to the level of globulin proteins present in the blood serum. Globulins are a group of proteins that are part of the blood plasma, along with albumin and fibrinogen. They are synthesized primarily in the liver and play various roles in the body's immune system, transport of substances, and blood clotting.

The measurement of serum globulin is often included in routine blood tests, such as a comprehensive metabolic panel (CMP) or a complete blood count (CBC). The serum globulin level is typically reported as part of the total protein measurement, which includes both albumin and globulin levels. The ratio of albumin to globulin (A/G ratio) can also be calculated from these values.

Normal serum globulin levels can vary depending on factors such as age, sex, and individual health status. In adults, the reference range for serum globulin is typically between 2.0 to 3.5 grams per deciliter (g/dL). However, reference ranges may differ between laboratories, so it's essential to interpret results in the context of the specific reference range provided by the testing facility.

Abnormalities in serum globulin levels can indicate various underlying health conditions, including:

- Liver Disease: Liver conditions such as hepatitis, cirrhosis, or liver failure can lead to alterations in serum globulin levels due to impaired synthesis or clearance of globulin proteins.

- Kidney Disease: Kidney disorders may affect serum globulin levels, particularly in cases of proteinuria (excessive protein in the urine) or impaired renal function.

- Inflammatory Conditions: Chronic inflammatory diseases, autoimmune disorders, and infections can cause elevated serum globulin levels as part of the body's immune response.

- Malnutrition: Severe malnutrition or protein deficiency may lead to decreased serum globulin levels, along with low total protein levels.

- Immunodeficiency Disorders: Certain immunodeficiency disorders or disorders affecting the production of immunoglobulin (antibodies) may result in abnormal serum globulin levels.

- Multiple Myeloma: Multiple myeloma, a type of blood cancer affecting plasma cells, can lead to elevated serum globulin levels due to the production of abnormal monoclonal proteins (M-proteins).

It's important to note that serum globulin levels are just one component of a comprehensive blood analysis and should be interpreted alongside other laboratory findings and clinical information to assess overall health and diagnose underlying conditions. If serum globulin levels are outside the normal range or if there are concerns about health status, further evaluation by a healthcare professional may be necessary for accurate diagnosis and management.

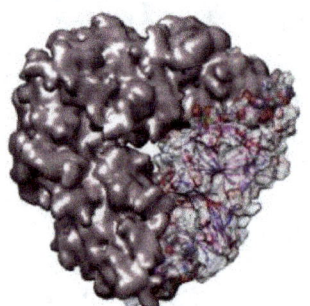

Total bilirubin is a measure of the total amount of bilirubin in the blood. Bilirubin is a yellowish pigment produced during the breakdown of red blood cells (hemoglobin). After red blood cells complete their life cycle, they are broken down in the spleen and liver, releasing hemoglobin. Hemoglobin is then converted into bilirubin in a series of enzymatic reactions.

There are two main forms of bilirubin in the blood:

- Indirect Bilirubin (Unconjugated Bilirubin): This form of bilirubin is insoluble in water and is bound to albumin for transport in the bloodstream from the liver to the liver. Indirect bilirubin is produced during the breakdown of hemoglobin in the spleen and liver.

- Direct Bilirubin (Conjugated Bilirubin): Once indirect bilirubin reaches the liver, it undergoes a chemical process called conjugation, where it is combined with glucuronic acid to form direct bilirubin. Direct bilirubin is water-soluble and can be excreted into bile for elimination from the body.

The total bilirubin level in the blood includes both indirect and direct bilirubin. It is typically measured as part of a comprehensive metabolic panel (CMP) or liver function tests (LFTs) and is reported in units such as milligrams per deciliter (mg/dL) or micromoles per liter (µmol/L).

Normal total bilirubin levels in adults are usually in the range of 0.3 to 1.2 mg/dL (5 to 21 µmol/L). However, reference ranges may vary slightly between laboratories.

Abnormal total bilirubin levels can indicate various health conditions, including:

- Liver Disorders: Conditions such as hepatitis, cirrhosis, liver cancer, or liver failure can cause elevated total bilirubin levels due to impaired bilirubin metabolism or excretion.

- Obstructive Jaundice: Blockages in the bile ducts, such as gallstones or tumors, can prevent the normal flow of bile and lead to an accumulation of conjugated bilirubin in the bloodstream, causing jaundice and elevated total bilirubin levels.

- Hemolytic Anemia: Increased breakdown of red blood cells (hemolysis) can result in elevated levels of indirect bilirubin due to the release of hemoglobin.

- Gilbert Syndrome: This benign genetic condition affects the liver's ability to process bilirubin, leading to mild elevation of indirect bilirubin levels without causing other symptoms.

- Drug Reactions: Certain medications or toxins can impair liver function and lead to elevated total bilirubin levels as a side effect.

- Newborn Jaundice: In newborns, transient jaundice is common due to the immature liver's inability to process bilirubin efficiently. This condition usually resolves on its own without treatment.

Monitoring total bilirubin levels can help diagnose and monitor liver and blood disorders. Abnormal results may prompt further evaluation, including additional blood tests, imaging studies, or liver biopsy, to determine the underlying cause and guide appropriate treatment. If total bilirubin levels are outside the normal range or if there are concerns about health status, individuals should consult with a healthcare professional for further evaluation and management.

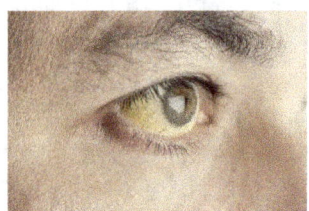

Alkaline phosphatase (ALP) is an enzyme found primarily in the liver, bones, kidneys, and bile ducts. It plays a role in various physiological processes, including bone formation, liver function, and bile production. Alkaline phosphatase is released into the bloodstream, where it can be measured through a blood test to assess liver and bone health.

Here's an overview of alkaline phosphatase and its significance:

- Physiological Functions:
- Bone Metabolism: Alkaline phosphatase is involved in bone mineralization and the formation of new bone tissue. It is produced by osteoblasts, the cells responsible for bone formation.

- Liver Function: Alkaline phosphatase is present in the liver, particularly in the bile ducts. It plays a role in bile production and the transport of bile acids, which are essential for digestion and the absorption of fats and fat-soluble vitamins.

- Other Tissues: Alkaline phosphatase is also found in other tissues, such as the kidneys, intestines, and placenta (during pregnancy). However, the liver and bones are the primary sources of alkaline phosphatase in the bloodstream.

- Blood Test:

Alkaline phosphatase levels can be measured through a blood test called an alkaline phosphatase assay. This test is often included as part of a comprehensive metabolic panel (CMP) or liver function tests (LFTs).

The normal range for alkaline phosphatase levels can vary depending on factors such as age, sex, and individual health status. In adults, the reference range is typically between 20 to 140 units per liter (U/L).

Elevated alkaline phosphatase levels may indicate liver or bone disorders, while low levels may be associated with malnutrition or certain genetic conditions.

- Clinical Significance:
- Liver Disorders: Elevated alkaline phosphatase levels may be observed in liver diseases such as hepatitis, cirrhosis, cholestasis (obstruction of bile flow), or liver cancer. Increased production of alkaline phosphatase by the liver or leakage of the enzyme into the bloodstream due to liver cell damage can lead to elevated levels.

- Bone Disorders: Alkaline phosphatase levels may also be elevated in conditions affecting bone metabolism, such as Paget's disease, osteomalacia, or bone metastases (cancer that has spread to the bones). Increased bone turnover or bone formation can lead to elevated alkaline phosphatase levels.

- Other Conditions: Elevated alkaline phosphatase levels may also be observed in conditions such as hyperparathyroidism, hyperthyroidism, vitamin D deficiency, or certain cancers.

Interpretation of alkaline phosphatase levels should be done in conjunction with other laboratory tests, clinical findings, and imaging studies to determine the underlying cause of abnormal results. If alkaline phosphatase levels are outside the normal range or if there are concerns about liver or bone health, individuals should consult with a healthcare professional for further evaluation and management.

Serum total bile acids (TBA) refer to the measurement of all bile acids present in the blood serum. Bile acids are natural substances synthesized by the liver from cholesterol and are critical for the digestion and absorption of fats and fat-soluble vitamins. Bile acids also play a role in the elimination of waste products, including excess cholesterol and toxins, from the body.

Here's an overview of serum total bile acids and their significance:

- Physiological Functions:
- Digestion and Absorption: Bile acids aid in the digestion and absorption of dietary fats in the small intestine. They emulsify fat globules, facilitating their breakdown by lipase enzymes into smaller particles that can be absorbed by intestinal cells.

- Micelle Formation: Bile acids form micelles, which are microscopic structures that solubilize and transport lipids, fat-soluble vitamins (A, D, E, and K), and cholesterol across the intestinal epithelium for absorption.

- Enterohepatic Circulation: Bile acids are reabsorbed in the ileum and transported back to the liver via the portal circulation in a process known as enterohepatic circulation. This recycling mechanism allows for efficient reuse of bile acids for digestion.

Blood Test:
- Measurement: Serum total bile acids can be measured through a blood test, typically performed as part of liver function tests or in the evaluation of cholestasis (impaired bile flow).
- Indications: Total bile acid levels in the blood may be elevated in conditions affecting liver function, bile duct obstruction, or disorders of bile acid metabolism.

Clinical Significance:

- Liver Diseases: Elevated serum total bile acids may indicate liver diseases such as hepatitis, cirrhosis, or liver cancer. Impaired liver function can lead to decreased bile acid synthesis or impaired bile secretion, resulting in elevated levels in the blood.

- Bile Duct Obstruction: Total bile acid levels may also be elevated in conditions causing obstruction of the bile ducts, such as gallstones, tumors, or strictures. Obstruction impedes the flow of bile into the intestine, leading to an accumulation of bile acids in the blood.

- Cholestasis: Cholestasis refers to impaired bile flow, either within the liver (intrahepatic) or in the bile ducts outside the liver (extra hepatic). Elevated total bile acids are a hallmark of cholestasis and may occur in conditions such as primary biliary cholangitis, primary sclerosing cholangitis, or drug-induced liver injury.

- Bile Acid Malabsorption: Decreased reabsorption of bile acids in the intestine can lead to increased excretion of bile acids in the feces (bile acid malabsorption) and compensatory synthesis of bile acids by the liver, resulting in elevated serum levels.

Interpretation of serum total bile acids levels should be done in conjunction with other laboratory tests, clinical findings, and imaging studies to determine the underlying cause of abnormal results. If serum total bile acids levels are outside the normal range or if there are concerns about liver or bile duct function, individuals should consult with a healthcare professional for further evaluation and management.

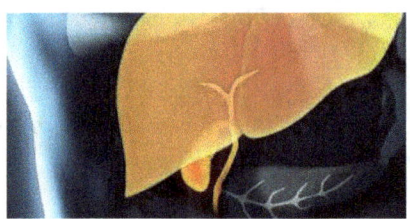

Bilirubin is a yellowish pigment produced during the breakdown of red blood cells (hemoglobin) in the liver. It is a waste product that is typically processed and excreted from the body through bile. Bilirubin is responsible for the yellow color of bruises and urine, and it is also the pigment responsible for the yellowing of the skin and eyes seen in jaundice.

Here are some key points about bilirubin:

- Formation: When red blood cells reach the end of their lifespan (about 120 days), they are broken down in the spleen and liver. Hemoglobin, the oxygen-carrying protein in red blood cells, is broken down into heme and globin. The heme portion is then converted into biliverdin, which is subsequently converted into bilirubin.

- Transport: Bilirubin is transported in the blood bound to albumin, a protein. This form of bilirubin is called unconjugated bilirubin or indirect bilirubin. In the bloodstream, bilirubin is carried to the liver.

- Processing in the Liver: In the liver, bilirubin undergoes a process called conjugation, where it is combined with glucuronic acid to make it water-soluble. This form of bilirubin is called conjugated bilirubin or direct bilirubin.

- Excretion: Conjugated bilirubin is excreted from the liver into the bile ducts and then into the intestines. In the intestines, bilirubin is further broken down by bacteria into urobilinogen, some of which is excreted in the feces, giving stool its characteristic brown color. Some urobilinogen is reabsorbed into the bloodstream and eventually excreted by the kidneys in the urine, giving it a yellow color.

- Measurement: Bilirubin levels can be measured in the blood to assess liver function and diagnose certain medical conditions. Total bilirubin measures both unconjugated and conjugated bilirubin, while direct bilirubin specifically measures conjugated bilirubin.

- Jaundice: Jaundice occurs when there is an accumulation of bilirubin in the body, leading to a yellowing of the skin and eyes. This can be caused by various factors, including liver disease, bile duct obstruction, excessive breakdown of red blood cells (hemolysis), or certain medications.

Bilirubin levels are typically reported in milligrams per deciliter (mg/dL) or micromoles per liter (µmol/L). Normal total bilirubin levels are typically between 0.3 to 1.2 mg/dL (5 to 21 µmol/L) in adults. Abnormal levels may indicate liver dysfunction, bile duct obstruction, or other medical conditions, and further evaluation may be needed to determine the underlying cause.

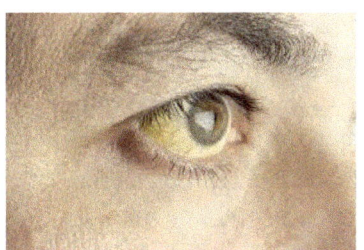

PANCREATIC FUNCTION

Insulin is a hormone produced by the pancreas that plays a key role in regulating blood sugar (glucose) levels in the body. It is secreted in response to elevated blood glucose levels, typically after a meal, and helps facilitate the uptake and storage of glucose by cells, particularly muscle, fat, and liver cells.

Here's how insulin works and its importance in the body:

- Glucose Uptake: When blood glucose levels rise after eating, specialized cells in the pancreas called beta cells detect the increase and release insulin into the bloodstream. Insulin acts as a signaling molecule, allowing glucose to enter cells from the bloodstream.

- Glycogen Synthesis: Once inside the cells, glucose can be used for immediate energy production or stored for future use. In muscle and liver cells, insulin promotes the synthesis of glycogen, a complex carbohydrate that serves as a storage form of glucose.

- Protein and Fat Synthesis: Insulin also stimulates the synthesis of proteins and fats in cells. In adipose tissue (fat cells), insulin promotes the uptake of glucose and the synthesis of fatty acids for storage as triglycerides. In muscle cells, insulin stimulates protein synthesis, which is important for muscle growth and repair.

- Inhibition of Glucose Production: Insulin inhibits the production of glucose in the liver (gluconeogenesis) by suppressing the release of glucose from glycogen stores and reducing the conversion of non-carbohydrate sources (such as amino acids and glycerol) into glucose.

- Regulation of Blood Sugar: Through its actions on glucose uptake, storage, and production, insulin helps maintain blood glucose levels within a narrow range, preventing hyperglycemia (high blood sugar) and hypoglycemia (low blood sugar).

- Role in Metabolism: Insulin is a central regulator of metabolism and energy balance in the body. Its actions on glucose, protein, and fat metabolism influence overall energy utilization, storage, and expenditure.

Insulin plays a critical role in the pathophysiology of diabetes mellitus, a group of metabolic disorders characterized by abnormal blood glucose regulation. In type 1 diabetes, the body's immune system mistakenly attacks and destroys the beta cells in the pancreas, leading to insulin deficiency. In type 2 diabetes, cells become resistant to the effects of insulin, requiring higher levels of insulin to maintain normal blood glucose levels.

Treatment for diabetes often involves insulin therapy, where individuals with type 1 diabetes or advanced type 2 diabetes may need to inject insulin to regulate their blood sugar levels. Additionally, lifestyle modifications, including dietary changes, exercise, and medications, may also be recommended to manage diabetes and improve insulin sensitivity.

Pancreatic polypeptide (PP) is a peptide hormone produced by specialized cells called F cells (or PP cells) located in the pancreas, specifically in the pancreatic islets (islets of Langerhans). PP secretion is primarily regulated by factors such as nutrient intake, particularly protein-rich meals, and fasting.

Here's an overview of pancreatic polypeptide and its functions:

- Regulation of Pancreatic Enzyme Secretion: Pancreatic polypeptide plays a role in regulating pancreatic enzyme secretion, particularly pancreatic bicarbonate secretion. It helps modulate the release of bicarbonate-rich pancreatic juice into the duodenum, which aids in neutralizing acidic chime (partially digested food) entering from the stomach.

- Appetite Regulation: Pancreatic polypeptide is involved in the regulation of appetite and food intake. It functions as a satiety hormone, meaning it helps signal to the brain that the body has consumed enough food, leading to a decrease in appetite and meal termination. PP levels typically rise after a meal, particularly in response to protein intake.

- Glucose Metabolism: While its role in glucose metabolism is less well understood compared to other pancreatic hormones like insulin and glucagon, pancreatic polypeptide may influence glucose homeostasis to some extent. Studies have suggested that PP may have an inhibitory effect on insulin secretion and may modulate glucose uptake and utilization in peripheral tissues.

- Gastrointestinal Motility: Pancreatic polypeptide has been implicated in the regulation of gastrointestinal motility, particularly in the small intestine. It may help modulate intestinal transit time and promote nutrient absorption by influencing smooth muscle activity in the gastrointestinal tract.

- Diagnostic Marker: Measurement of pancreatic polypeptide levels in the blood can serve as a diagnostic marker for certain medical conditions. Elevated PP levels may be observed in conditions such as pancreatic neuroendocrine tumors (pancreatic NETs), also known as pancreatic islet cell tumors or pancreatic endocrine tumors.

Overall, pancreatic polypeptide plays diverse roles in regulating pancreatic function, appetite, gastrointestinal motility, and glucose metabolism. Its secretion is tightly regulated in response to various physiological stimuli, and abnormalities in PP levels may be associated with certain medical conditions. However, further research is needed to fully elucidate the mechanisms and clinical significance of pancreatic polypeptide in human health and disease.

Glucagon is a peptide hormone produced by alpha cells in the pancreas, which are located in clusters known as the islets of Langerhans. It plays a crucial role in glucose metabolism and helps regulate blood sugar levels, primarily by increasing blood glucose concentration when it falls too low.

Here's an overview of glucagon and its functions:

- Counter regulatory Hormone: Glucagon acts as a counter regulatory hormone to insulin. While insulin helps lower blood sugar levels by promoting glucose uptake and storage, glucagon works to raise blood sugar levels when they fall below normal levels, ensuring a constant supply of glucose to the body's cells.

- Glycogenolysis: Glucagon stimulates the breakdown of glycogen, a stored form of glucose found in the liver and muscles, into glucose molecules. This process, known as glycogenolysis, releases glucose into the bloodstream, thereby increasing blood sugar levels.

- Gluconeogenesis: Glucagon promotes gluconeogenesis, the synthesis of glucose from non-carbohydrate sources such as amino acids, lactate, and glycerol. It stimulates the liver to convert these substrates into glucose, providing an additional source of glucose to maintain blood sugar levels.

- Lipolysis: In addition to its effects on glucose metabolism, glucagon also stimulates lipolysis, the breakdown of triglycerides stored in adipose tissue into fatty acids and glycerol. These fatty acids can serve as alternative fuel sources for tissues such as muscle and the liver during periods of low blood sugar.

- Protein Catabolism: Glucagon can also promote protein catabolism, particularly in the liver, where it stimulates the breakdown of proteins into amino acids. These amino acids can then be used as substrates for gluconeogenesis to generate glucose.

- Regulation of Blood Sugar: Glucagon secretion is primarily regulated by blood glucose levels. When blood sugar levels drop (such as during fasting or between meals), glucagon secretion is stimulated to raise blood glucose levels.

Conversely, when blood sugar levels rise (such as after a meal), insulin secretion increases, and glucagon secretion decreases.

- Stress Response: Glucagon also plays a role in the body's stress response by mobilizing energy reserves to meet increased energy demands during stressful situations.

Overall, glucagon plays a critical role in maintaining glucose homeostasis by stimulating the release of glucose from glycogen stores, promoting gluconeogenesis, and mobilizing energy reserves. Dysregulation of glucagon secretion or action can contribute to disorders of glucose metabolism, such as diabetes mellitus. Consequently, medications that target glucagon signaling are used in the management of diabetes to help regulate blood sugar levels.

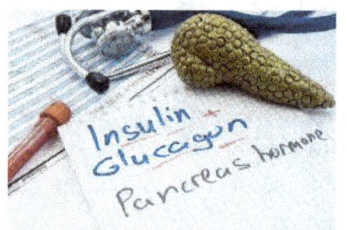

KIDNEY FUNCTION

The urobilinogen index is a measure used in urine analysis to assess the levels of urobilinogen present in the urine. Urobilinogen is a breakdown product of bilirubin, which is formed during the breakdown of hemoglobin in the liver.

The urobilinogen index is calculated by comparing the concentration of urobilinogen in the urine sample to the urine creatinine concentration. Creatinine is a waste product generated from the breakdown of creatine in muscles and is excreted at a relatively constant rate in urine. By normalizing the urobilinogen concentration to creatinine, variations in urine concentration due to factors such as hydration status are taken into account.

The formula for calculating the urobilinogen index is as follows:

Urobilinogen index=Urobilinogen concentration in urine (mg/dL)Urine creatinine concentration (mg/dL)Urobilinogen index=Urine creatinine concentration (mg/dL)Urobilinogen concentration in urine (mg/dL)

The urobilinogen index is typically expressed in units of mg/g creatinine.

The urobilinogen index is used in the evaluation of liver function and the diagnosis of liver diseases such as hepatitis, cirrhosis, and obstructive jaundice. Elevated levels of urobilinogen in urine may indicate increased breakdown of red blood cells, liver dysfunction, or bile duct obstruction. Conversely, low levels of urobilinogen in urine may be observed in conditions such as liver failure or biliary tract obstruction. However, it's important to interpret the urobilinogen index in the context of other clinical findings and laboratory tests to determine the underlying cause of abnormal results.

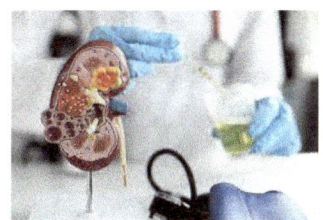

Uric acid is a waste product produced during the breakdown of purines, which are compounds found in certain foods and also produced by the body. Most uric acid is dissolved in the blood and excreted from the body through the kidneys in the urine. Abnormal levels of uric acid can be indicative of various health conditions, including gout, kidney disease, and metabolic disorders.

Here's a brief overview of uric acid measurement and its significance:
- Blood Uric Acid: Blood uric acid levels can be measured through a blood test. The reference range for uric acid levels in the blood may vary depending on the laboratory, but generally, normal levels fall within the range of 2.5 to 7.0 mg/dL for males and 1.5 to 6.0 mg/dL for females. Elevated blood uric acid

levels (hyperuricemia) may be associated with conditions such as gout, kidney disease, dehydration, certain medications, and dietary factors.

- Urine Uric Acid: Uric acid levels can also be measured in urine. Abnormal levels of uric acid in urine may indicate conditions such as kidney stones, kidney disease, or metabolic disorders.

- Uric Acid Crystals: When uric acid levels are too high, they can form crystals in the joints, leading to a painful condition known as gout. Uric acid crystals can also form kidney stones when they accumulate in the kidneys.

- Risk Factors: Several factors can contribute to high uric acid levels, including genetics, diet (consumption of purine-rich foods such as red meat, seafood, and alcohol), obesity, certain medications (such as diuretics and aspirin), and underlying health conditions (such as hypertension, diabetes, and metabolic syndrome).

It's important to note that while uric acid levels are a useful indicator in diagnosing and managing certain medical conditions, they are only one piece of the puzzle. A comprehensive assessment, including medical history, physical examination, and other laboratory tests, is necessary for accurate diagnosis and treatment. If you have concerns about your uric acid levels or related symptoms, it's best to consult with a healthcare professional for proper evaluation and management

The Blood Urea Nitrogen (BUN) test measures the level of urea nitrogen in the blood. It is a common blood test used to evaluate kidney function and assess the body's nitrogen balance. Urea is a waste product formed when the liver breaks down proteins, and it is excreted by the kidneys through urine.

The BUN test is often ordered as part of a comprehensive metabolic panel (CMP) or basic metabolic panel (BMP) to:

- Assess Kidney Function: The kidneys filter urea from the blood and excrete it in the urine. Elevated BUN levels can indicate impaired kidney function or decreased glomerular filtration rate (GFR), which may occur in conditions such as acute or chronic kidney disease.

- Monitor Treatment: BUN levels may be monitored in patients with kidney disease or undergoing dialysis to assess the effectiveness of treatment and evaluate disease progression.

- Evaluate Dehydration: Dehydration or decreased fluid intake can cause an increase in BUN levels due to decreased urine output and concentration of urea in the blood.

The BUN test measures the concentration of urea nitrogen in the blood and is reported in units such as milligrams per deciliter (mg/dL) or mill moles per liter (mmol/L). The normal range for BUN levels may vary depending on factors such as age, gender, and individual health status. However, typical reference ranges are approximately 7 to 20 mg/dL (2.5 to 7.1 mmol/L) in adults.

It's important to interpret BUN levels in conjunction with other kidney function tests, such as serum creatinine levels and estimated glomerular filtration rate (eGFR), as well as clinical findings and medical history. Abnormal BUN levels may indicate kidney dysfunction, dehydration, urinary tract obstruction, heart failure, liver disease, or other medical conditions. If BUN levels are outside the normal range or if there are concerns about kidney function, further evaluation and consultation with a healthcare professional may be necessary.

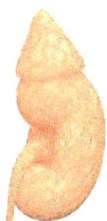
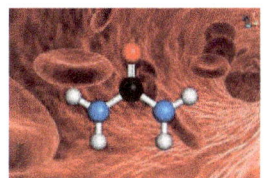

Proteinuria is the presence of an abnormal amount of protein in the urine. The proteinuria index is not a standardized term, but it may refer to various methods used to quantify the amount of protein excreted in the urine or to assess the severity of proteinuria. *Here are some ways proteinuria can be evaluated:*

- Urinary Protein Concentration: Proteinuria can be quantified by measuring the concentration of protein in a urine sample, typically reported in milligrams per deciliter (mg/dL) or grams per liter (g/L). This method provides a quantitative measure of protein excretion but does not account for variations in urine volume.

- Urinary Protein-to-Creatinine Ratio (UPCR): The UPCR is a commonly used method to assess proteinuria, particularly in clinical practice and research settings. It involves measuring both urinary protein and urinary creatinine levels and expressing the ratio of protein to creatinine. This ratio helps normalize protein excretion to urine concentration and corrects for variations in urine volume. The UPCR is typically reported in units such as milligrams of protein per gram of creatinine (mg/g) or grams of protein per mole of creatinine (g/mol).

- 24-Hour Urine Protein: In some cases, proteinuria may be assessed by collecting urine over a 24-hour period and measuring the total amount of protein excreted during that time. This method provides a more accurate assessment of protein excretion than a spot urine sample and is often used in research studies or when precise quantification of proteinuria is necessary.

- Dipstick Urinalysis: Dipstick urinalysis is a rapid and convenient method used to screen for proteinuria in clinical practice. Urine dipstick tests detect the presence of protein in urine based on chemical reactions. The results are semi-quantitative and are typically reported as negative, trace, 1+, 2+, 3+, or 4+ depending on the concentration of protein detected.

The presence and severity of proteinuria can provide valuable information about kidney function and underlying health conditions. Proteinuria may be transient and benign, or it may indicate kidney disease, systemic disorders, or other medical conditions. Depending on the cause and severity of proteinuria, further evaluation, monitoring, and treatment may be necessary. If proteinuria is detected, it is important to consult with a healthcare professional for proper assessment and management.

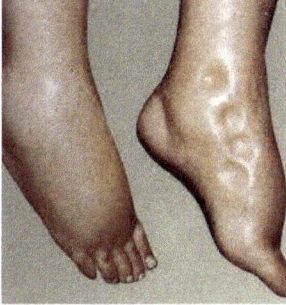

LUNG FUNCTION

Vital capacity (VC) is a measure of the maximum amount of air that can be forcibly exhaled from the lungs after a maximum inhalation. It represents the total volume of air that can be moved in and out of the lungs during a respiratory cycle and is an important indicator of lung function.

Here's how vital capacity is typically measured and its significance:

- Measurement: Vital capacity is measured using a device called a spirometer, which records the volume of air exhaled during a forced expiration maneuver. The individual inhales deeply and then exhales forcefully and completely into the spirometer as quickly as possible until no more air can be expelled. The volume of air exhaled during this maneuver is measured in liters (L) or milliliters (mL) and represents the vital capacity.

- Components: Vital capacity is composed of three primary lung volumes:
- Inspiratory Reserve Volume (IRV): The maximum amount of air that can be inhaled beyond the normal tidal volume.

- Tidal Volume (TV): The volume of air breathed in and out during normal, relaxed breathing.

- Expiratory Reserve Volume (ERV): The maximum amount of air that can be exhaled beyond the normal tidal volume.

Mathematically, vital capacity can be expressed as the sum of these three volumes:
$$VC = IRV + TV + ERV$$

- Significance: Vital capacity reflects the overall lung function and respiratory muscle strength. It can be affected by various factors, including age, gender, height, body composition, and lung health. Reduced vital capacity may indicate lung diseases such as chronic obstructive pulmonary disease (COPD), asthma, restrictive lung diseases, or neuromuscular disorders. Monitoring changes in vital capacity over time can help assess disease progression, response to treatment, and overall respiratory health.

- Clinical Application: Vital capacity measurements are commonly used in pulmonary function tests (PFTs) to assess lung function and diagnose respiratory disorders. Spirometer, which includes the measurement of vital capacity, is often performed as a routine screening test in clinical settings, occupational health assessments, and sports medicine evaluations.

- Normal Range: The normal range for vital capacity can vary widely among individuals and is influenced by factors such as age, sex, height, and ethnicity. In adults, the average vital capacity is approximately 3 to 5 liters for males and 2 to 4 liters for females. However, individual values may fall outside this range due to differences in lung size, respiratory muscle strength, and overall health status.

Overall, vital capacity is an essential measure of lung function that provides valuable information about respiratory health and helps in the diagnosis and management of various respiratory conditions.

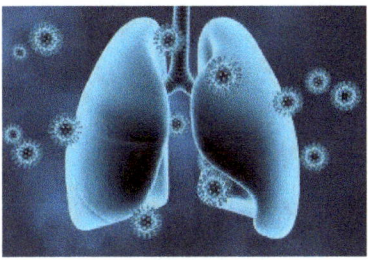

Total lung capacity (TLC) is the maximum volume of air that the lungs can hold after maximal inhalation. *It represents the sum of all lung volumes and is composed of several components:*

- Inspiratory Reserve Volume (IRV): The additional volume of air that can be inhaled beyond the normal tidal volume during maximal inspiration.

- Tidal Volume (TV): The volume of air breathed in and out during normal, relaxed breathing.

- Expiratory Reserve Volume (ERV): The additional volume of air that can be exhaled beyond the normal tidal volume during maximal expiration.

- Residual Volume (RV): The volume of air remaining in the lungs after maximal expiration. This volume cannot be measured directly using spirometer but can be estimated using specialized lung function tests such as body plethysmography.

Mathematically, total lung capacity can be expressed as the sum of these volumes:

$$TLC = IRV + TV + ERV + RV$$

Total lung capacity varies among individuals and is influenced by factors such as age, sex, height, body composition, and lung health. TLC tends to increase with age until early adulthood and then gradually decreases with age due to changes in lung elasticity and respiratory muscle strength.

Total lung capacity measurements are essential in assessing overall lung function and diagnosing various respiratory disorders, including obstructive lung diseases (such as chronic obstructive pulmonary disease, asthma) and restrictive lung diseases (such as pulmonary fibrosis, sarcoidosis). Changes in TLC may indicate abnormalities in lung volume, compliance, or airway obstruction, and can help guide treatment decisions and monitor disease progression.

Total lung capacity is typically measured using pulmonary function tests (PFTs), which may include spirometer, lung volumes, and diffusing capacity tests. Spirometer alone does not measure total lung capacity directly but provides valuable information about lung function and can be used in conjunction with other tests to assess respiratory health comprehensively.

Overall, total lung capacity serves as a fundamental parameter in evaluating lung function and plays a crucial role in diagnosing and managing respiratory diseases.

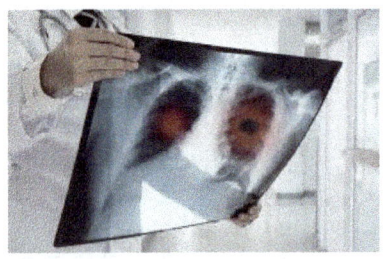
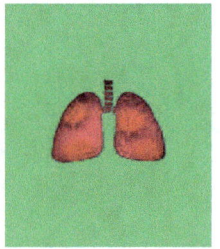

Airway resistance refers to the resistance encountered by the flow of air through the airways during breathing. It is a measure of the impedance to airflow within the respiratory system and is influenced by various factors, including the size and condition of the airways, lung compliance, and the viscosity of the air.

Here's a closer look at airway resistance and its significance:

- Physiology: Airway resistance primarily occurs in the conducting airways of the respiratory system, including the trachea, bronchi, and bronchioles. Resistance to airflow is mainly determined by the diameter of the airways, with smaller airways offering greater resistance than larger ones. Smooth muscle tone within the airways, as well as factors such as mucus secretion and airway inflammation, can also affect airway resistance.

- Measurement: Airway resistance is typically measured using pulmonary function tests (PFTs) such as spirometer and body plethysmography. Specific parameters, such as airway resistance (Raw) and specific airway resistance (sRaw), may be calculated or derived from these tests to quantify the resistance to airflow within the respiratory system. Raw is measured in units such as centimeters of water per liter per second ($cmH_2O/L/s$) or in millimeters of mercury per liter per second ($mmHg/L/s$).

- Clinical Significance: Abnormalities in airway resistance can indicate underlying respiratory conditions, such as asthma, chronic obstructive pulmonary disease (COPD), bronchitis, or bronchiolitis. Increased airway resistance may result from airway constriction, inflammation, or narrowing due to factors such as bronchospasm, mucosal edema, mucus accumulation, or structural changes in the airway walls. Decreased airway resistance may occur in conditions such as emphysema or when airway patency is improved through bronchodilator therapy.

- Treatment: Management of airway resistance depends on the underlying cause. In conditions characterized by increased resistance, bronchodilators (such as beta-agonists or anticholinergic) may be used to relax airway smooth muscle and alleviate bronchoconstriction. Anti-inflammatory medications (such as corticosteroids) may also be prescribed to reduce airway inflammation and improve airflow. In severe cases, mechanical ventilation or other advanced respiratory support measures may be necessary to maintain adequate ventilation.

- Monitoring: Monitoring airway resistance over time can help assess disease progression, evaluate treatment efficacy, and guide therapeutic interventions. Changes in airway resistance may reflect improvements or exacerbations in respiratory function and can inform adjustments to the treatment regimen.

Overall, understanding airway resistance is essential in the assessment and management of respiratory disorders and plays a critical role in optimizing lung function and respiratory health.

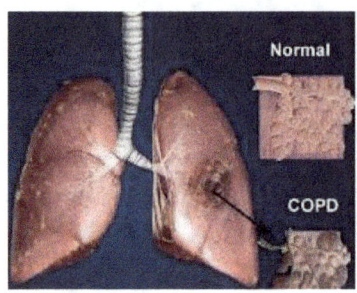

Arterial oxygen content refers to the amount of oxygen dissolved in arterial blood per unit volume. It is a crucial parameter in assessing the oxygen-carrying capacity of the blood and the adequacy of oxygen delivery to tissues throughout the body.

Arterial oxygen content is influenced by several factors, including the partial pressure of oxygen (PaO2), hemoglobin concentration (Hb), and the oxygen saturation of hemoglobin (SaO2). The oxygen content of arterial blood can be calculated using the following formula:

$$CaO2 = (1.34 \times Hb \times SaO2) + (0.003 \times PaO2) \quad CaO2 = (1.34 \times Hb \times SaO2) + (0.003 \times PaO2)$$

Where:

CaO2CaO2= Arterial oxygen content (in mL of O2 per deciliter of blood)

1.34 = Oxygen-carrying capacity of hemoglobin (in mL of O2 per gram of hemoglobin)

Hb = Hemoglobin concentration (in grams per deciliter)

SaO2 = Oxygen saturation of hemoglobin (expressed as a decimal, ranging from 0 to 1)

0.003 = Solubility coefficient of oxygen in blood plasma (in mL of O2 per mmHg per deciliter)

PaO2 = Partial pressure of oxygen in arterial blood (in mmHg)

The first term of the equation represents the oxygen content bound to hemoglobin (oxygen saturation), while the second term represents the dissolved oxygen content in the plasma.

Arterial oxygen content is essential for maintaining cellular metabolism and tissue oxygenation. Changes in arterial oxygen content can occur in various conditions, including respiratory disorders (such as pneumonia, asthma, or chronic obstructive pulmonary disease), cardiovascular diseases (such as heart failure or cyanotic heart defects), anemia, altitude exposure, and during mechanical ventilation.

In clinical practice, arterial blood gas (ABG) analysis is commonly performed to measure arterial blood oxygenation parameters, including PaO_2, SaO_2, and pH. These measurements, along with the calculated arterial oxygen content, help assess respiratory function, oxygenation status, and acid-base balance in patients with respiratory and cardiovascular diseases, as well as those undergoing anesthesia or critical care management.

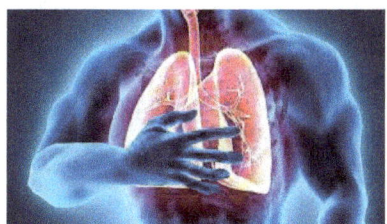

BRAIN NERVE

The status of brain tissue blood supply is crucial for maintaining normal brain function and preventing neurological damage. The brain requires a constant and adequate supply of oxygen and nutrients delivered through cerebral blood flow (CBF) to support its metabolic demands.

Here are some key points regarding the status of brain tissue blood supply:

- Cerebral Blood Flow (CBF): Cerebral blood flow refers to the volume of blood that perfuses the brain per unit of time. It is tightly regulated to meet the metabolic demands of brain tissue and maintain cerebral homeostasis. CBF is influenced by factors such as cerebral perfusion pressure (CPP), vascular resistance, and auto regulation mechanisms.

- Auto regulation: The brain has intrinsic mechanisms to regulate its blood flow over a range of systemic blood pressures to ensure consistent perfusion. This auto regulatory mechanism helps maintain a relatively stable CBF despite fluctuations in systemic blood pressure. However, severe changes in blood pressure outside the auto regulatory range can lead to cerebral hypo perfusion or hyper perfusion, potentially causing ischemia or cerebral edema, respectively.

- Vascular Anatomy: The brain receives its blood supply from two main arterial systems: the anterior circulation, primarily supplied by the internal carotid arteries, and the posterior circulation, primarily supplied by the vertebral arteries. These arteries give rise to smaller branches that form an extensive network of cerebral blood vessels, including arteries, arterioles, capillaries, venules, and veins.

- Cerebral Perfusion Pressure (CPP): CPP is the pressure gradient that drives blood flow to the brain and is calculated as the difference between mean arterial pressure (MAP) and intracranial pressure (ICP). Maintaining an adequate CPP is essential for ensuring sufficient blood flow to meet the metabolic demands of brain tissue while preventing cerebral ischemia or hypoxia.

- Regulation of Cerebral Blood Flow: CBF is regulated by various factors, including metabolic demand, arterial blood gases (such as oxygen and carbon dioxide levels), neural activity, and autonomic nervous system control. These factors influence cerebral vascular tone, diameter, and resistance, thereby modulating CBF to match metabolic needs.

- Monitoring: Monitoring the status of brain tissue blood supply is essential in clinical practice, particularly in the management of conditions such as traumatic brain injury, stroke, intracranial hemorrhage, and cerebral ischemia. Techniques such as trans cranial Doppler ultrasound, cerebral oximetry, and invasive monitoring of ICP and CPP are commonly used to assess CBF, oxygenation, and cerebral perfusion in critically ill patients.

Overall, maintaining adequate cerebral blood flow and perfusion is vital for preserving brain function and preventing neurological injury. Monitoring and managing factors that affect cerebral blood supply are critical aspects of patient care in neurocritical care settings.

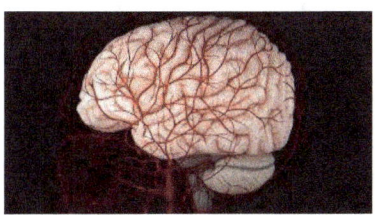

Cerebral arteriosclerosis, also known as cerebrovascular arteriosclerosis or cerebral small vessel disease, refers to a condition characterized by thickening, hardening, and narrowing of the small arteries and arterioles in the brain. It is a type of arteriosclerosis that affects the blood vessels supplying the brain, leading to impaired blood flow and potential damage to brain tissue.

Here are some key points about cerebral arteriosclerosis:

- Pathophysiology: Cerebral arteriosclerosis typically results from the accumulation of fatty deposits, cholesterol, calcium, and other substances (atherosclerosis) in the walls of small arteries and arterioles in the brain. These deposits can cause the blood vessels to become stiff, narrow, or occluded, reducing blood flow to affected areas of the brain. Chronic hypertension, dyslipidemia, diabetes, smoking, and aging are among the common risk factors associated with the development and progression of cerebral arteriosclerosis.

- Clinical Manifestations: Cerebral arteriosclerosis can lead to various neurological symptoms and cognitive impairments, depending on the severity and location of the affected blood vessels. *Common manifestations may include*:

- Cognitive decline
- Memory loss
- Mood changes
- Gait disturbances
- Balance problems

- Transient ischemic attacks (TIAs) or mini-strokes
- Lacunar infarcts (small, deep-seated strokes)
- Subcortical vascular dementia
- Intracerebral hemorrhage

- Imaging Findings: Imaging studies such as magnetic resonance imaging (MRI) or computed tomography (CT) scans may reveal characteristic findings associated with cerebral arteriosclerosis, including:

White matter hyper intensities (WMHs) on T2-weighted MRI, indicating areas of ischemic damage or demyelination in the brain's white matter.

Lacunes or small infarcts in subcortical regions of the brain, resulting from occlusion of small penetrating arteries.

Micro bleeds or hemosiderin deposits, indicating small areas of bleeding within the brain tissue.

Enlarged perivascular spaces (Virchow-Robin spaces), reflecting changes in brain vasculature due to chronic arteriosclerosis.

- Management and Prevention: Treatment strategies for cerebral arteriosclerosis aim to control underlying risk factors, optimize cardiovascular health, and prevent further vascular damage. This may include lifestyle modifications (e.g., smoking cessation, regular exercise, and healthy diet), management of hypertension and dyslipidemia with medications, and antiplatelet therapy (e.g., aspirin) to reduce the risk of stroke. Additionally, managing comorbid conditions such as diabetes and atrial fibrillation is essential for preventing complications associated with cerebral arteriosclerosis.

Overall, cerebral arteriosclerosis is a chronic condition associated with progressive damage to the brain's small blood vessels, leading to cognitive decline, stroke, and other neurological complications. Early detection, risk factor modification, and appropriate medical management are crucial for optimizing outcomes and reducing the risk of complications in affected individuals.

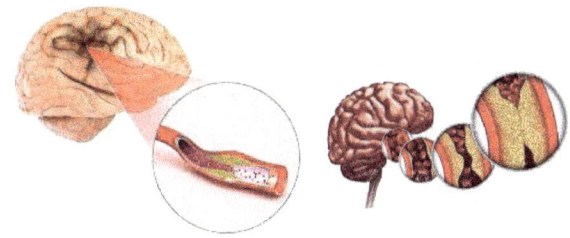

Cranial nerves are a set of twelve pairs of nerves that emerge directly from the brain and primarily innervate structures within the head and neck region. Each cranial nerve serves specific functions related to sensory, motor, or autonomic innervation of various structures, including muscles, glands, and sensory receptors.

Here's a brief overview of the functional status of each cranial nerve:

- Olfactory Nerve (CN I):
- Function: Sense of smell (olfaction).
- Assessment: Evaluate the ability to detect and identify different odors.
- Optic Nerve (CN II):
- Function: Vision.
- Assessment: Visual acuity, visual field testing, pupillary reflexes, and fundoscopic examination.
- Oculomotor Nerve (CN III):

- Function: Innervates extra ocular muscles controlling eye movements (except lateral rectus and superior oblique), as well as the pupillary sphincter muscle.
- Assessment: Assess eye movements, pupillary size, reaction to light (pupillary light reflex), accommodation reflex, and eyelid position.

Trochlear Nerve (CN IV):

- Function: Innervates the superior oblique muscle, which controls downward and inward eye movements.
- Assessment: Evaluate eye movements, particularly downward and inward gaze.

Trigeminal Nerve (CN V):

- Function: Sensation of the face, scalp, oral cavity, and teeth; motor innervation to the muscles of mastication.
- Assessment: Test sensation in different areas of the face, corneal reflex, and assess motor function by testing jaw movements and muscle strength.

Abducens Nerve (CN VI):

- Function: Innervates the lateral rectus muscle, which controls outward eye movement (abduction).
- Assessment: Evaluate eye movements, particularly lateral gaze.

Facial Nerve (CN VII):

- Function: Controls facial expression muscles, taste sensation from the anterior two-thirds of the tongue, and lacrimation and salivation.
- Assessment: Assess facial symmetry, strength of facial muscles, taste sensation, and ability to close the eyes tightly and wrinkle the forehead.

Vestibulocochlear Nerve (CN VIII):

- Function: Hearing (cochlear branch) and balance and spatial orientation (vestibular branch).
- Assessment: Audiometry for hearing, Romberg test, and vestibular function testing.

Glossopharyngeal Nerve (CN IX):

- Function: Sensation of the posterior one-third of the tongue, taste sensation from the posterior one-third of the tongue, sensation from the pharynx, and innervation of the stylopharyngeus muscle involved in swallowing.
- Assessment: Evaluate gag reflex, taste sensation, and sensation in the throat.

Vagus Nerve (CN X):

- Function: Innervates muscles of the pharynx and larynx involved in swallowing and phonation, sensation from the larynx, and parasympathetic innervation to thoracic and abdominal organs.
- Assessment: Assess swallowing function, voice quality, and evaluate for any signs of autonomic dysfunction.

Accessory Nerve (CN XI):

- Function: Controls the sternocleidomastoid and trapezius muscles, involved in head and shoulder movement.
- Assessment: Test muscle strength and coordination of head and shoulder movements.

Hypoglossal Nerve (CN XII):

- Function: Innervates the muscles of the tongue, involved in speech articulation and swallowing.
- Assessment: Evaluate tongue movement, strength, and coordination.

Assessment of cranial nerve function is an essential component of the neurological examination and can provide valuable information about the integrity of the nervous system and potential underlying neurological conditions. Dysfunction of one or more cranial nerves may indicate peripheral nerve injury, cranial nerve lesions, or central nervous system pathology, requiring further evaluation and management by a healthcare professional.

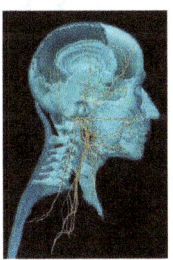

There are several techniques and measures used in cognitive neuroscience to study emotional processing and **sentiment in the brain**. *These measures include*:

- Functional Magnetic Resonance Imaging (fMRI): Functional MRI is a neuroimaging technique that measures changes in blood flow and oxygenation levels in the brain. It is commonly used to investigate brain regions involved in emotional processing by comparing brain activity during the presentation of emotional stimuli (such as images or videos) with neutral stimuli. Analysis of fMRI data can identify brain regions associated with emotional responses and assess their connectivity patterns.

- Electroencephalography (EEG): EEG measures electrical activity generated by neurons in the brain using electrodes placed on the scalp. EEG studies can assess brain responses to emotional stimuli with high temporal resolution, allowing researchers to identify event-related potentials (ERPs) associated with emotional processing. ERPs, such as the P300 or late positive potential (LPP), are components of the EEG signal that reflect cognitive and emotional processing of stimuli.

- Magneto encephalography (MEG): MEG is a neuroimaging technique that measures the magnetic fields generated by neuronal activity in the brain. Similar to EEG, MEG provides high temporal resolution and is used to study the timing and dynamics of brain responses to emotional stimuli.

- Functional Near-Infrared Spectroscopy (fNIRS): fNIRS measures changes in blood oxygenation levels in the brain using near-infrared light. It is a non-invasive technique that can assess brain activity associated with emotional processing, particularly in regions near the surface of the cortex.

- Behavioral Measures: Alongside neuroimaging techniques, behavioral measures such as self-report questionnaires, emotion recognition tasks, or physiological measures (e.g., heart rate variability) are used to assess subjective experiences of emotion and sentiment.

By combining these techniques, researchers can investigate the neural correlates of emotional experiences, identify brain regions involved in emotional processing, and explore individual differences in emotional responses. Understanding the neural basis of sentiment and emotion has implications for various fields, including psychology, psychiatry, and neurology, and can contribute to the development of interventions for mood disorders and mental health conditions.

Memory function, there are several standardized tests and cognitive assessments commonly used to evaluate different aspects of memory.

Here are some commonly used memory assessments:

- Verbal Memory Tests: These tests assess an individual's ability to remember verbal information, such as lists of words or stories. Examples include the Rey Auditory Verbal Learning Test (RAVLT) and the California Verbal Learning Test (CVLT).

- Visual Memory Tests: Visual memory tests evaluate an individual's ability to remember visual information, such as geometric figures, faces, or spatial layouts. Examples include the Rey-Osterrieth Complex Figure Test and the Visual Reproduction subtest of the Wechsler Memory Scale.

- Working Memory Tasks: Working memory refers to the temporary storage and manipulation of information for cognitive tasks. Tests of working memory assess an individual's ability to hold and manipulate information in mind. Examples include digit span tasks and the n-back task.

- Episodic Memory Tests: Episodic memory involves the recollection of specific events or experiences from one's past. Tests of episodic memory assess an individual's ability to remember autobiographical events or details from specific episodes. Examples include autobiographical memory interviews and recall of personally experienced events.

- Semantic Memory Tests: Semantic memory refers to general knowledge about the world, concepts, and facts. Tests of semantic memory assess an individual's ability to remember general knowledge and factual information. Examples include tests of vocabulary knowledge and general knowledge quizzes.

- Prospective Memory Tests: Prospective memory involves remembering to perform intended actions or tasks in the future. Tests of prospective memory assess an individual's ability to remember to carry out planned actions at specific times or in specific contexts. Examples include time-based and event-based prospective memory tasks.

These memory assessments may be administered individually or as part of a comprehensive neuropsychological evaluation to assess memory function in clinical and research settings. Performance on memory tests can provide valuable information about cognitive abilities, identify memory deficits associated with neurological conditions or brain injuries, and inform treatment planning and interventions

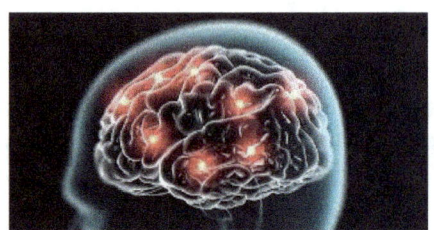

BONE MINERAL DENSITY

The osteoclast coefficient is a measurement used to quantify the activity and effectiveness of osteoclasts in the process of bone restoration. Osteoclasts are specialized cells that break down and resorb bone tissue, playing a key role in bone remodeling and turnover. The osteoclast coefficient is typically calculated by measuring the rate of bone restoration and comparing it to the number and activity of osteoclasts present in the bone tissue. A higher osteoclast coefficient indicates increased bone restoration activity, which can be associated with conditions such as osteoporosis, rheumatoid arthritis, and other bone diseases.

Monitoring the osteoclast coefficient can help in assessing bone health and identifying potential issues related to bone restoration. Treatments for conditions involving abnormal bone restoration may target osteoclast activity to help restore bone density and prevent fractures. The amount of calcium lost refers to the quantity of calcium that is removed from the body through various means, such as urine, feces, or sweat. Calcium is a crucial mineral that plays a vital role in bone health, muscle function, nerve transmission, and other physiological processes.

The body tightly regulates calcium levels through a process called calcium homeostasis, which involves the balance between calcium absorption, storage, and excretion. When there is an imbalance in this process, it can lead to either too much calcium being lost or retained in the body.

Excessive calcium loss can occur due to various factors, such as inadequate dietary intake, certain medical conditions (such as hyperparathyroidism or kidney disease), medications, or hormonal imbalances. Chronic calcium loss can lead to weakened bones, increased risk of fractures, muscle cramps, and other health problems.

Monitoring the amount of calcium lost can be important in evaluating overall calcium balance and bone health. Treatment strategies to address excessive calcium loss may include dietary changes, supplementation, medication, and management of underlying medical conditions. It is always recommended to consult with a healthcare provider for personalized advice and guidance on managing calcium levels.

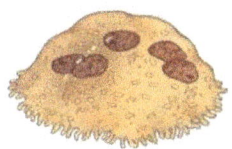

Bone hyperplasia, also known as osteoporosis or marble bone disease, is a rare genetic disorder characterized by the abnormal thickening or increased density of bones. This condition can result in weakened bones that are prone to fractures, as well as other complications such as impaired bone marrow function and nerve compression.

The degree of bone hyperplasia can vary among individuals and is typically assessed through imaging studies such as X-rays, CT scans, or bone density tests. These tests can help evaluate the extent of bone thickening, areas affected, and the overall impact on bone structure and function.

Treatment for bone hyperplasia may focus on managing symptoms, preventing fractures, and addressing complications associated with the condition. This can include medications to help with bone resorption, physical therapy, and in severe cases, bone marrow transplants or surgery.

Monitoring the degree of bone hyperplasia is essential for assessing disease progression, response to treatment, and overall bone health. Regular follow-up with healthcare providers, including bone specialists or genetic counselors, can help in managing the condition and improving quality of life for individuals affected by bone hyperplasia.

Disorder characterized by increased bone density and abnormal bone growth. In osteoporosis, there is a defect in the osteoclasts, the cells responsible for breaking down bone tissue, leading to impaired bone restoration and bone remodeling.

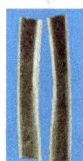

The degree of bone hyperplasia in osteoporosis can vary depending on the specific genetic mutation involved and the severity of the condition. In some cases, individuals with osteoporosis may have mild symptoms and minimal bone dysplasia, while others may experience more significant bone overgrowth and density.

Radiographic imaging, such as X-rays or CT scans, can help assess the degree of bone hyperplasia and provide information about the bone structure and density. Features commonly observed in osteoporosis include a "marble bone" appearance on imaging, thickened bones, and reduced bone marrow spaces.

Treatment for osteoporosis is focused on managing symptoms and complications of the disease. This may include supportive care, such as physical therapy, pain management, and treatment of fractures. In some cases, bone marrow transplantation or other specialized therapies may be considered.

The degree of bone hyperplasia in osteoporosis can impact the progression and management of the condition, so close monitoring and multidisciplinary care involving specialists in genetics, orthopedics, and endocrinology are essential for optimal outcomes.

The degree of osteoporosis is typically assessed using bone density measurements, often through a dual-energy X-ray absorptiometry (DXA) scan. This scan measures bone mineral density (BMD) and compares it to the average BMD of healthy young adults, generating a T-score. The T-score indicates how much your bone density differs from the average young adult.

The World Health Organization (WHO) defines osteoporosis based on T-scores:

Normal: T-score above -1.

Osteopenia (low bone mass): T-score between -1 and -2.5.

Osteoporosis: T-score -2.5 or below.

The severity of osteoporosis can further be categorized based on fracture risk and other factors. It's essential to consult a healthcare professional for an accurate assessment and appropriate management plan if you have concerns about osteoporosis.

Bone mineral density (BMD) is a measure of the amount of mineral content, such as calcium and phosphorus, in a certain volume of bone tissue. It is a critical indicator of bone strength and quality.

BMD is typically measured using a dual-energy X-ray absorptiometry (DXA) scan, which provides a T-score indicating how your bone density compares to that of a healthy young adult population. As mentioned earlier:

- A T-score above -1 is considered normal.
- A T-score between -1 and -2.5 indicates osteopenia (low bone mass).
- A T-score of -2.5 or below signifies osteoporosis.

BMD can also be measured at different sites of the body, such as the hip, spine, or forearm, as these areas are most commonly affected by osteoporosis-related fractures.

Maintaining healthy bone mineral density is crucial for overall bone health and reducing the risk of fractures, especially as one ages. Regular exercise, a balanced diet rich in calcium and vitamin D, and avoidance of factors that contribute to bone loss (such as smoking and excessive alcohol consumption) can help maintain or improve bone density. If you have concerns about your bone health, it's essential to consult with a healthcare professional for personalized advice and management.

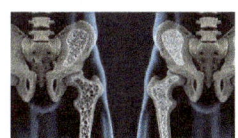

RHEUMATOID ARTHRITIS

Cervical calcification typically refers to the presence of calcium deposits within the cervical spine, which are the vertebrae in the neck region. These calcifications can occur for various reasons, including degenerative changes, injury, or conditions such as cervical spondylitis.

The degree of cervical calcification can vary depending on factors such as the extent of calcium deposition, the size of the deposits, and whether they are causing symptoms or complications. Imaging studies such as X-rays, CT scans, or MRIs may be used to assess the degree and extent of calcification.

The severity of cervical calcification and its impact on health can vary widely among individuals. In some cases, cervical calcification may be asymptomatic and require no specific treatment. However, if the calcifications are causing symptoms such as neck pain, stiffness, or neurological symptoms like weakness or numbness in the arms or hands, further evaluation and management may be necessary.

Treatment options for symptomatic cervical calcification may include medications for pain management, physical therapy, lifestyle modifications, and in some cases, surgical intervention to alleviate pressure on the spinal cord or nerve roots.

It's essential to consult with a healthcare professional for an accurate diagnosis and appropriate management plan if you have concerns about cervical calcification or are experiencing symptoms related to it.

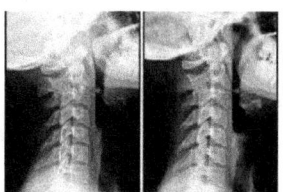

Lumber calcification refers to calcium deposits in the lumbar spine, the lower portion of the vertebral column.

Calcification in the lumbar spine can occur due to various reasons, including degenerative changes, injury, or conditions such as osteoarthritis or spinal stenosis. The degree of lumbar calcification can vary depending on factors such as the extent of calcium deposition, the size of the deposits, and whether they are causing symptoms or complications.

Imaging studies such as X-rays, CT scans, or MRIs may be used to assess the degree and extent of calcification in the lumbar spine.

The severity of lumbar calcification and its impact on health can vary among individuals. In some cases, lumbar calcification may be asymptomatic and require no specific treatment. However, if the calcifications are causing symptoms such as back pain, stiffness, or neurological symptoms like weakness or numbness in the legs, further evaluation and management may be necessary.

Treatment options for symptomatic lumbar calcification may include medications for pain management, physical therapy, lifestyle modifications, and in some cases, surgical intervention to alleviate pressure on the spinal cord or nerve roots.

It's essential to consult with a healthcare professional for an accurate diagnosis and appropriate management plan if you have concerns about lumbar calcification or are experiencing symptoms related to it, which refers to an abnormal increase in the number of bone cells or bone tissue.

Hyperplasia is a term used in biology to describe the proliferation or increase in the number of cells in a tissue or organ beyond what is typically considered normal. In the context of bone, hyperplasia could refer to conditions such as osteoporosis (excessive bone density due to abnormal bone growth), osteoblastoma (benign bone tumor), or other conditions characterized by excessive bone formation.

The coefficient part of the term suggests a quantitative measure or ratio associated with this hyperplasia, but without further context or definition, it's challenging to provide specific information.

If you have a specific context or further details about what you're referring to, please provide them, and I'll do my best to assist you. Otherwise, if you have concerns about bone health or specific medical conditions, it's essential to consult with a healthcare professional for accurate diagnosis and guidance.

Various indices or scores used in the assessment and diagnosis of osteoporosis.

Here are a few key measurements and indicators commonly used in evaluating osteoporosis:

- T-score: This score compares a person's bone density to that of a healthy young adult of the same gender. It's typically measured using a DXA scan and is expressed in standard deviations (SD) from the average. A T-score of -2.5 or lower indicates osteoporosis.

- Z-score: Similar to the T-score, but it compares bone density to that of individuals of the same age, gender, and ethnicity. A Z-score significantly below average may indicate secondary causes of bone loss.

- FRAX®: The Fracture Risk Assessment Tool calculates a person's 10-year probability of a major osteoporotic fracture (including hip, spine, forearm, or shoulder fractures) and hip fracture alone. It takes into account various risk factors, including age, sex, weight, height, prior fracture history, parental hip fracture history, smoking status, glucocorticoid use, rheumatoid arthritis, alcohol intake, and secondary osteoporosis.

Bone Mineral Density (BMD): This is measured using a DXA scan and represents the amount of mineral in bone tissue. Low BMD is associated with an increased risk of fractures and osteoporosis.

Trabecular Bone Score (TBS): TBS is a measurement obtained from DXA images that assesses the microarchitecture of bone. It provides additional information about fracture risk beyond BMD alone.

These are some of the common tools and measurements used in the evaluation of osteoporosis risk and bone health. If you're referring to a specific coefficient or index, please provide more context, and I can offer further assistance. Additionally, consulting with a healthcare professional is important for proper evaluation and management of osteoporosis.

Various blood tests or biomarkers used in the diagnosis and management of rheumatic conditions such as rheumatoid arthritis (RA) or systemic lupus erythematous (SLE).

In rheumatoid arthritis, for example, various blood tests are commonly used to aid in diagnosis and monitoring disease activity. *Some of the key blood tests include:*

- Rheumatoid Factor (RF): RF is an antibody that is often elevated in individuals with rheumatoid arthritis. However, it can also be present in other conditions and in healthy individuals.

- Anti-cyclic citrullinated peptide (anti-CCP) antibodies: These antibodies are more specific to rheumatoid arthritis and are often used in conjunction with RF testing for diagnosis.

- C-reactive protein (CRP) and erythrocyte sedimentation rate (ESR): These are markers of inflammation that can be elevated in various rheumatic conditions, including rheumatoid arthritis, lupus, and others. They are not specific to rheumatoid arthritis but can be helpful in assessing disease activity.

- Antinuclear antibodies (ANA): ANA testing is used in the diagnosis of autoimmune diseases such as systemic lupus erythematous (SLE) and other connective tissue disorders.

- Complete blood count (CBC): A CBC with differential can provide information about white blood cell counts, red blood cell counts, and platelet counts, which may be abnormal in various rheumatic conditions.

These are just a few examples of blood tests commonly used in the evaluation of rheumatic diseases. If you have a specific context or are referring to a particular test or measurement, please provide more information, and I can offer further assistance. Additionally, consulting with a healthcare professional is important for proper evaluation and management of rheumatic conditions.

BONE GROWTH INDEX

Bone alkaline phosphatase (BAP) is an enzyme produced primarily by osteoblasts, which are cells responsible for bone formation. BAP plays a crucial role in bone mineralization by regulating the deposition of calcium and phosphate ions during bone formation. It is released into the bloodstream during the process of bone remodeling.

Measurement of bone alkaline phosphatase levels in the blood can provide insight into bone metabolism and turnover. Elevated levels of BAP may indicate increased bone formation, such as in conditions like Paget's disease of bone or during periods of rapid bone growth, such as adolescence or pregnancy. Conversely, low levels of BAP may suggest decreased bone formation, as seen in osteomalacia or osteoporosis.

Bone alkaline phosphatase levels are often measured through a blood test. It's important to interpret BAP levels in conjunction with other clinical information and additional tests, such as bone density measurements, to assess bone health comprehensively.

If you have concerns about your bone health or specific medical conditions, it's essential to consult with a healthcare professional for proper evaluation and management

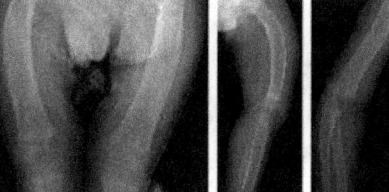

Osteocalcin is a protein that is produced by osteoblasts, the cells responsible for bone formation. It plays a crucial role in bone mineralization, which is the process of incorporating calcium and other minerals into the bone matrix to make bones strong and rigid.

Osteocalcin is often used as a marker of bone formation and turnover. Blood levels of osteocalcin can indicate the rate of bone formation, with higher levels typically associated with increased bone turnover. Measurement of osteocalcin levels is often included in tests assessing bone health, such as those used in the diagnosis and monitoring of osteoporosis.

In addition to its role in bone health, osteocalcin has also been implicated in other physiological processes, including regulation of glucose metabolism and energy expenditure. It is considered a hormone that may influence metabolism and energy homeostasis.

Overall, osteocalcin serves as an important biomarker for bone health and may have broader implications in metabolic processes beyond bone metabolism. If you have concerns about your bone health or specific medical conditions, it's essential to consult with a healthcare professional for proper evaluation and management

The healing process of long bones typically involves several stages:

- Inflammatory Phase: This begins immediately after the bone is fractured and lasts for several days. Blood vessels at the fracture site constrict to minimize bleeding, and inflammatory cells, such as neutrophils and macrophages, migrate to the area to remove debris and initiate the healing process.

- Reparative Phase: This phase lasts for several weeks and involves the formation of a soft callus composed of fibrous tissue and cartilage around the fracture site. Osteoblasts, which are bone-forming cells, migrate to the area and begin to produce new bone tissue.

- Hard Callus Formation: Over the next several weeks to months, the soft callus is gradually replaced by a hard callus made of woven bone, which provides structural support to the healing bone.

- Bone Remodeling: This final phase can last for months to years, during which the hard callus is gradually remodeled into mature lamellar bone. This process involves the removal of excess bone tissue and the restoration of the bone's original shape and strength.

The status of long bone healing can vary depending on factors such as the severity of the fracture, the individual's overall health, and the effectiveness of treatment. Imaging studies such as X-rays or CT scans are often used to monitor the progress of bone healing and assess the stability of the fracture site.

In general, if the healing process is proceeding as expected, signs of bone union, such as the formation of a visible callus and evidence of bone remodeling, will be observed on imaging studies. However, if there are complications such as delayed union, nonunion, or maluion, additional interventions may be necessary to promote healing and restore function to the affected limb.

If you have concerns about the healing status of a long bone fracture, it's essential to consult with a healthcare professional, such as an orthopedic surgeon, who can evaluate your specific situation and recommend appropriate treatment options

The healing process of cartilage in short bones, or any bone for that matter, is more complex and challenging compared to other tissues like skin or muscle. Cartilage is a specialized connective tissue with limited blood supply and cellular activity, which makes its healing capacity relatively poor compared to other tissues.

When cartilage in short bones is injured, such as in a fracture involving the cartilaginous portions, *the healing process typically involves the following steps:*

- Inflammatory Phase: Similar to bone healing, the initial response involves an inflammatory reaction at the site of injury. Blood vessels near the injured area dilate, allowing immune cells to migrate to the site and initiate the removal of damaged tissue.

- Repair Phase: Cartilage repair is more limited compared to other tissues due to its avascular nature and low cellularity. Repair processes in cartilage involve the migration of chondrocytes (cartilage cells) to the injured area, where they attempt to produce new extracellular matrix (ECM) components to fill the defect. However, the repair is often incomplete, and the newly formed tissue may not fully restore the original structure and function of the cartilage.

- Remodeling Phase: Over time, the newly formed tissue undergoes remodeling, which involves further organization and maturation of the ECM. However, the regenerated tissue may lack the structural integrity and mechanical properties of healthy cartilage.

Overall, cartilage healing in short bones is limited and often leads to the formation of fibrocartilage, which is a less specialized type of cartilage compared to the hyaline cartilage found in healthy joints. This fibrocartilage may be less resistant to mechanical stress and more prone to degeneration over time.

Treatment options for cartilage injuries in short bones may include conservative measures such as rest, physical therapy, and pain management, as well as surgical interventions such as arthroscopic debridement, micro fracture, autologous chondrocyte implantation (ACI), or osteochondral auto graft transplantation (OATS). However, complete restoration of cartilage function and structure remains a significant challenge in clinical practice.

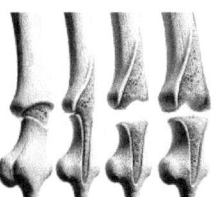

The epiphyseal line, also known as the epiphyseal plate or growth plate, is a thin line of cartilage that appears in the bones of children and adolescents, particularly in the long bones such as the femur, tibia, and humorous. It exists at the junction between the diaphysis (shaft) and the epiphysis (end) of the bone.

During childhood and adolescence, this plate is responsible for longitudinal bone growth, as it allows for the lengthening of bones. As a child grows, new bone is formed on the epiphyseal side while cartilage is replaced by bone tissue on the diaphysis side. This process continues until the individual reaches skeletal maturity, at which point the epiphyseal plate disappears and is replaced by a bony structure called the epiphyseal line.

Once the epiphyseal line forms, the bone can no longer grow in length, and the individual has reached their adult height. The presence of the epiphyseal line indicates that the bones have stopped growing longitudinally.

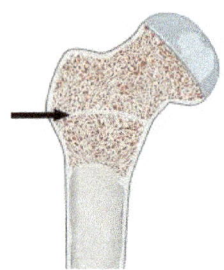

BLOOD SUGAR

The coefficient of insulin secretion typically refers to a measure of the rate or efficiency at which insulin is secreted by the pancreas in response to various stimuli, such as glucose levels in the blood.

Insulin secretion is a complex process regulated by multiple factors, including blood glucose levels, other hormones such as glucagon, amino acids, fatty acids, neural inputs, and more. The coefficient of insulin secretion may be influenced by genetic factors, lifestyle, diet, and certain medical conditions.

Researchers and clinicians may use different methods to assess insulin secretion, such as insulin secretion rate calculations during glucose tolerance tests, measurement of fasting insulin levels, or more sophisticated techniques involving intravenous glucose tolerance tests combined with mathematical modeling.

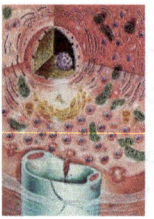
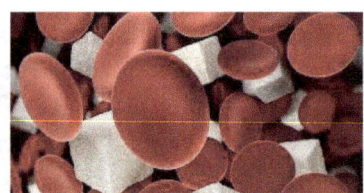

Understanding the coefficient of insulin secretion can be crucial in diagnosing and managing conditions like diabetes mellitus, where abnormalities in insulin secretion can lead to deregulated blood sugar levels and associated complications.

- Insulin Sensitivity Coefficient: This coefficient, often denoted as "SI" (for sensitivity index), is a measure of how effectively the body's tissues respond to insulin in lowering blood sugar levels. It's used in mathematical models to assess insulin sensitivity and insulin resistance, which are key factors in conditions like type 2 diabetes.

- Glycemic Variability Coefficient: This coefficient may refer to a measure of how much blood sugar levels fluctuate over time. It could be calculated using standard deviation, coefficient of variation, or other statistical methods applied to blood glucose data obtained from continuous glucose monitoring (CGM) devices or periodic blood glucose measurements.

If you have a specific context in mind or more details about what you're referring to with "blood sugar coefficient," feel free to provide them, and I can offer more tailored information.

The term "**urine sugar coefficient**" likely refers to a measure or ratio used in the context of urinalysis to assess the presence of sugar (glucose) in urine, which is a condition known as glycosuria. Glycosuria can occur in various medical conditions, such as uncontrolled diabetes mellitus or renal tubular disorders.

The urine sugar coefficient could be calculated by comparing the concentration of glucose in urine to the concentration of glucose in the blood. This comparison helps evaluate how effectively the kidneys are reabsorbing glucose from the filtrate during the process of urine formation. Normally, the kidneys reabsorb almost all of the glucose from the filtrate back into the bloodstream, so the presence of glucose in urine suggests either an excess of glucose in the blood (as seen in uncontrolled diabetes) or impaired renal glucose reabsorption.

The coefficient could be expressed as a ratio (e.g., urine glucose concentration divided by blood glucose concentration) or as a percentage. Higher values of the urine sugar coefficient indicate more significant glycosuria.

It's important to note that the presence of glucose in urine can also be influenced by factors such as the renal threshold for glucose, renal function, hydration status, and certain medications. Therefore, the interpretation of the urine sugar coefficient should be done in conjunction with other clinical information to determine the underlying cause. If you have specific concerns about your urine sugar levels, it's best to consult with a healthcare professional for proper evaluation and management.

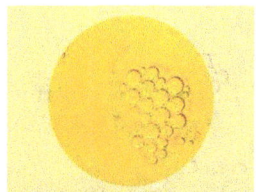

TRACE ELEMENTS

Calcium is a mineral that plays a crucial role in various physiological processes throughout the body. It's perhaps best known for its role in maintaining the health of bones and teeth, but it's also involved in muscle function, nerve transmission, hormone secretion, and blood clotting.

Here are some key points about calcium:

- Bone Health: Calcium is a major component of bone tissue, contributing to bone strength and structure. Adequate calcium intake throughout life, along with other bone-supporting nutrients like vitamin D and magnesium, is important for building and maintaining healthy bones, thereby reducing the risk of osteoporosis and fractures.

- Muscle Function: Calcium ions are necessary for muscle contraction. When a muscle is stimulated, calcium is released from storage sites within the muscle cells, triggering the contraction process. After the muscle contraction, calcium is pumped back into storage to relax the muscle.

- Nerve Function: Calcium ions play a role in transmitting nerve impulses throughout the body. They are involved in the release of neurotransmitters, which are chemical messengers that allow nerve cells to communicate with each other.

- Blood Clotting: Calcium is essential for the blood clotting process. When a blood vessel is injured, platelets (blood cells) adhere to the site of injury and release chemical signals that lead to the formation of a blood clot. Calcium ions help facilitates several steps in this process, ultimately leading to the formation of a stable clot to stop bleeding.

- Other Functions: Calcium also plays a role in various other biological processes, including enzyme activation, cell signaling, and hormone secretion.

It's important to consume adequate amounts of calcium through diet or supplementation to support these functions. Good dietary sources of calcium include dairy products (such as milk, yogurt, and cheese), leafy green vegetables (such as kale and broccoli), fortified foods (such as fortified plant-based milks and cereals), and certain nuts and seeds. The recommended daily intake of calcium varies by age, sex, and other factors, but generally ranges from 1000 to 1300 milligrams per day for adults.

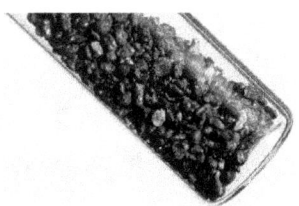

Iron is an essential mineral that plays several important roles in the body:
- Oxygen Transport: Iron is a key component of hemoglobin, the protein in red blood cells that carries oxygen from the lungs to tissues throughout the body. Hemoglobin binds to oxygen in the lungs, and then releases it to cells in need of oxygen for energy production. Iron is also a component of myoglobin, a

protein found in muscle cells that stores and transports oxygen for muscle function.

- Energy Production: Iron is a component of several enzymes involved in energy metabolism. These enzymes are essential for the production of adenosine triphosphate (ATP), the molecule that provides energy for cellular processes.

- Immune Function: Iron is necessary for proper functioning of the immune system. It is involved in the proliferation and differentiation of immune cells, and plays a role in the production of certain immune factors.

- Brain Function: Iron is important for normal brain development and function. It is involved in the synthesis of neurotransmitters such as dopamine, norepinephrine, and serotonin, which are important for mood regulation, cognition, and behavior.

- DNA Synthesis: Iron is required for the synthesis of DNA, the genetic material found in all cells. It is a component of enzymes involved in DNA replication and repair.

Iron deficiency can lead to a condition called iron deficiency anemia, characterized by low levels of hemoglobin and red blood cells, resulting in symptoms such as fatigue, weakness, shortness of breath, pale skin, and decreased exercise tolerance. Iron deficiency anemia is one of the most common nutritional deficiencies worldwide.

Good dietary sources of iron include red meat, poultry, fish, beans, lentils, tofu, fortified cereals, spinach, and other leafy green vegetables. Consuming iron-rich foods along with sources of vitamin C can enhance iron absorption. In some cases, iron supplements may be recommended to treat or prevent iron deficiency. However, excessive iron intake can be harmful, so it's important to follow recommended guidelines for iron supplementation.

Zinc is an essential mineral that plays a crucial role in numerous biological processes throughout the body. *Here are some key functions of zinc:*

- Immune Function: Zinc is vital for a healthy immune system. It is involved in the development and function of immune cells, including T cells, B cells, and natural killer cells. Zinc deficiency can impair immune responses, making individuals more susceptible to infections.

- Wound Healing: Zinc is necessary for proper wound healing. It plays a role in cell division, cell growth, and tissue repair. Zinc deficiency can delay wound healing and increase the risk of infections.

- DNA Synthesis and Cell Division: Zinc is required for the synthesis of DNA, RNA, and proteins. It is essential for cell division, growth, and repair. Zinc deficiency can lead to impaired growth and development, particularly in children.

- Sensory Perception: Zinc is important for the function of taste and smell receptors. Zinc deficiency can lead to alterations in taste and smell perception.

- Hormone Regulation: Zinc is involved in the synthesis, storage, and secretion of various hormones, including insulin, thyroid hormones, and sex hormones. It helps regulate hormone levels and supports reproductive health.

- Antioxidant Activity: Zinc acts as an antioxidant, helping to protect cells from oxidative damage caused by free radicals. It helps neutralize free radicals and reduce oxidative stress.

- Skin Health: Zinc plays a role in maintaining the health of the skin and mucous membranes. It supports skin integrity, reduces inflammation, and helps in the treatment of conditions such as acne and eczema.

Good dietary sources of zinc include red meat, poultry, fish, shellfish, dairy products, nuts, seeds, legumes, and whole grains. The recommended daily intake of zinc varies by age, sex, and life stage, but for most adults, it ranges from 8 to 11 milligrams per day. Zinc supplements may be recommended for individuals at risk of deficiency, such as pregnant or lactating women, vegetarians, or those with certain medical conditions that affect zinc absorption or metabolism. However, excessive intake of zinc can be harmful, so it's important to follow recommended guidelines for supplementation.

Selenium is an essential trace mineral that plays important roles in various physiological processes in the body. Here are some key functions of selenium:

Antioxidant Activity: Selenium is a component of selenoproteins, which are enzymes that act as antioxidants. These enzymes help protect cells from damage caused by free radicals and oxidative stress. Selenium works in concert with other antioxidants like vitamin E to neutralize free radicals and reduce the risk of chronic diseases such as cardiovascular disease and cancer.

- Thyroid Function: Selenium is required for the synthesis and metabolism of thyroid hormones. It is a component of enzymes involved in the conversion of thyroxine (T4) to triiodothyronine (T3), the active form of thyroid hormone. Adequate selenium levels are important for maintaining thyroid function and regulating metabolism.

- Immune Function: Selenium plays a role in supporting the immune system. It helps regulate the production and activity of immune cells and cytokines, which are signaling molecules involved in immune responses. Selenium deficiency has been associated with impaired immune function and increased susceptibility to infections.

- Reproductive Health: Selenium is important for male and female reproductive health. It is involved in spermatogenesis (sperm production) and sperm motility in men, and it plays a role in the protection of eggs from oxidative damage in women. Adequate selenium levels may also support fertility and pregnancy outcomes.

- Cognitive Function: Selenium may have neuroprotective effects and contribute to cognitive function. Some research suggests that selenium deficiency may be associated with cognitive decline and neurological disorders such as Alzheimer's disease.

- Anticancer Effects: Selenium has been studied for its potential role in cancer prevention. Some research suggests that selenium may help reduce the risk of certain cancers, particularly prostate, lung, colorectal, and bladder cancers. However, the evidence is mixed, and more research is needed to understand the relationship between selenium and cancer risk.

Good dietary sources of selenium include seafood (such as fish, shellfish, and crustaceans), Brazil nuts, organ meats, meat, poultry, eggs, dairy products, and certain grains and vegetables (depending on the selenium content of the soil). The recommended daily intake of selenium varies by age, sex, and life stage, but for most adults, it ranges from 55 to 70 micrograms per day. Supplementation with selenium may be appropriate for individuals at risk of deficiency, but excessive intake can be harmful, so it's important to follow recommended guidelines for supplementation.

Phosphorus is an essential mineral that plays several critical roles in the body's physiology and metabolism. *Here are some key functions of phosphorus:*

- Bone and Teeth Health: Phosphorus is a major component of bones and teeth, providing strength and structure. Along with calcium, phosphorus forms calcium phosphate crystals, which make up the mineral matrix of bones and teeth. Adequate phosphorus intake is essential for maintaining healthy bone density and preventing conditions like osteoporosis.

- Energy Metabolism: Phosphorus is a component of adenosine triphosphate (ATP), the primary energy currency of cells. ATP stores and transfers energy within cells, powering various cellular processes, including muscle contraction, nerve signaling, and biochemical reactions involved in metabolism.

- Cellular Structure and Function: Phosphorus is a key component of cell membranes, where it helps form phospholipids, which are essential for maintaining membrane integrity and facilitating cell signaling. Phosphorus is also involved in DNA and RNA synthesis, playing a crucial role in genetic expression and cellular replication.

- Acid-Base Balance: Phosphorus plays a role in maintaining acid-base balance in the body. Phosphates act as buffers, helping to regulate pH levels in bodily fluids and prevent excessive acidity or alkalinity.

- Kidney Function: Phosphorus levels in the body are regulated by the kidneys, which help excrete excess phosphorus through urine. Disorders affecting kidney function can lead to disturbances in phosphorus balance, potentially resulting in hypophosphatemia (high blood phosphorus levels) or hypophosphatemia (low blood phosphorus levels).

- Muscle Function: Phosphorus is involved in muscle contraction and relaxation. It helps regulate calcium levels within muscle cells, which are critical for muscle function. Phosphorus deficiency can impair muscle function and lead to weakness and fatigue.

- Nerve Function: Phosphorus plays a role in nerve signaling and neurotransmitter release. It helps maintain the electrical potential across cell membranes, which is essential for nerve impulse transmission.

Good dietary sources of phosphorus include dairy products (such as milk, cheese, and yogurt), meat, poultry, fish, eggs, nuts, seeds, legumes, and whole grains. The recommended daily intake of phosphorus varies by age, sex, and life stage, but for most adults, it ranges from 700 to 1250 milligrams per day. While phosphorus deficiency is rare in healthy individuals with a balanced diet, excessive phosphorus intake from supplements or processed foods can have adverse health effects, particularly in individuals with kidney disease. Therefore, it's important to consume phosphorus in moderation and as part of a well-rounded diet.

Potassium is an essential mineral and electrolyte that plays a vital role in numerous physiological processes in the human body. *Here are some key functions of potassium:*

- Fluid and Electrolyte Balance: Potassium helps regulate fluid balance within cells and maintains proper electrolyte balance in the body. It works in conjunction with sodium to regulate fluid levels and control blood pressure.

- Muscle Function: Potassium is crucial for normal muscle function, including muscle contraction and relaxation. It helps transmit nerve impulses to muscle cells, allowing them to contract in response to stimuli. Potassium deficiency can lead to muscle weakness, cramps, and spasms.

- Heart Function: Potassium is essential for maintaining normal heart rhythm and function. It helps regulate the electrical activity of the heart and is involved in generating the electrical impulses that coordinate heartbeats. Adequate potassium intake is important for preventing arrhythmias and maintaining cardiovascular health.

- Blood Pressure Regulation: Potassium plays a role in blood pressure regulation by counteracting the effects of sodium. It helps relax blood vessel walls, which can lower blood pressure. Diets high in potassium and low in sodium are associated with a reduced risk of hypertension and cardiovascular disease.

- Kidney Function: Potassium is involved in kidney function and helps regulate the balance of fluids and electrolytes in the body. The kidneys play a critical role in maintaining potassium balance by excreting excess potassium through urine. Disorders affecting kidney function can lead to potassium imbalances.

- Bone Health: While calcium and phosphorus are the primary minerals involved in bone health, potassium also plays a role in maintaining bone density and strength. Some research suggests that diets high in potassium may help reduce the risk of osteoporosis and bone fractures.

- Acid-Base Balance: Potassium helps maintain acid-base balance in the body by acting as a buffer to neutralize acids. It helps regulate pH levels in bodily fluids, preventing excessive acidity or alkalinity.

Good dietary sources of potassium include fruits (such as bananas, oranges, and avocados), vegetables (such as spinach, potatoes, and tomatoes), legumes, nuts, seeds, dairy products, fish, and lean meats. The recommended daily intake of potassium varies by age, sex, and life stage, but for most adults, it ranges from 2000 to 3500 milligrams per day. It's important to consume an adequate amount of potassium through diet to support overall health and prevent potassium deficiency, which can have serious health consequences. However, excessive potassium intake from supplements can also be harmful, particularly for individuals with certain medical conditions such as kidney disease. Therefore, it's best to obtain potassium from food sources and consult with a healthcare provider before taking potassium supplements.

Magnesium is an essential mineral that plays numerous crucial roles in the human body. *Here are some key functions of magnesium:*

- Muscle Function: Magnesium is involved in muscle contraction and relaxation. It helps regulate the activity of muscle cells by influencing calcium transport across cell membranes. Adequate magnesium levels are necessary for proper muscle function, including heart muscle function.

- Nervous System Function: Magnesium plays a role in nerve transmission and neuromuscular conduction. It helps regulate the release of neurotransmitters and is involved in maintaining the electrical potentials of nerve cells. Magnesium deficiency can lead to neurological symptoms such as muscle spasms, tremors, and seizures.

- Energy Metabolism: Magnesium is a cofactor for numerous enzymes involved in energy metabolism. It participates in the synthesis of adenosine triphosphate (ATP), the primary energy currency of cells, and helps regulate the activity of enzymes involved in glycolysis, the tricarboxylic acid (TCA) cycle, and oxidative phosphorylation.

- Protein Synthesis: Magnesium is required for the synthesis of proteins, including enzymes, structural proteins, and regulatory proteins. It is involved in the activation of amino acids and the formation of peptide bonds during protein synthesis.

- Bone Health: Magnesium plays a role in bone formation and mineralization. It helps regulate the activity of osteoblasts (cells that build bone) and osteoclasts (cells that break down bone), contributing to bone remodeling and maintenance of bone density. Adequate magnesium intake is important for preventing osteoporosis and maintaining bone health.

- Heart Health: Magnesium is important for maintaining normal heart rhythm and function. It helps regulate the contraction of cardiac muscle cells and supports the electrical activity of the heart. Magnesium deficiency has been associated with an increased risk of arrhythmias, hypertension, and cardiovascular disease.

- Blood Glucose Regulation: Magnesium plays a role in insulin secretion and glucose metabolism. It helps facilitate the uptake of glucose into cells and is involved in the activation of enzymes that regulate glucose utilization. Magnesium deficiency may impair insulin sensitivity and contribute to the development of insulin resistance and type 2 diabetes.

Good dietary sources of magnesium include green leafy vegetables (such as spinach and kale), nuts and seeds (such as almonds, cashews, and pumpkin seeds), legumes, whole grains, avocados, bananas, and dark chocolate. The recommended daily intake of magnesium varies by age, sex, and life stage, but for most adults, it ranges from 300 to 400 milligrams per day. While magnesium deficiency is relatively rare in healthy individuals with a balanced diet, certain factors such as gastrointestinal disorders, kidney disease, and certain medications can increase the risk of magnesium deficiency. In such cases, supplementation may be necessary under the guidance of a healthcare provider.

Copper is an essential trace mineral that plays various important roles in the human body. *Here are some key functions of copper:*

- Enzyme Cofactor: Copper serves as a cofactor for numerous enzymes involved in a wide range of biological processes. These enzymes are involved in cellular energy production (such as cytochrome c oxidase in the electron transport chain), antioxidant defense (such as superoxide dismutase), neurotransmitter synthesis, connective tissue formation, and iron metabolism.

- Iron Metabolism: Copper is involved in the absorption, transport, and metabolism of iron. It helps convert iron into a form that can be transported in the blood (ferrous iron to ferric iron) and incorporated into hemoglobin, the protein in red blood cells that carries oxygen. Copper deficiency can lead to impaired iron utilization and iron-deficiency anemia.

- Connective Tissue Formation: Copper is essential for the synthesis of collagen and elastin, two proteins that are critical for the structure and integrity of connective tissues, including skin, blood vessels, bones, and tendons. Copper deficiency can impair connective tissue formation and lead to symptoms such as joint pain and skin abnormalities.

- Neurotransmitter Synthesis: Copper is involved in the synthesis of neurotransmitters such as dopamine, norepinephrine, and epinephrine. These neurotransmitters play important roles in mood regulation, stress response, and cognitive function. Copper deficiency may affect neurotransmitter levels and contribute to neurological symptoms such as depression and anxiety.

- Pigment Production: Copper is involved in the synthesis of melanin, the pigment that gives color to skin, hair, and eyes. It plays a role in melanin production by serving as a cofactor for the enzyme tyrosine, which is involved in the conversion of tyrosine to melanin. Copper deficiency may lead to alterations in skin and hair pigmentation.

- Immune Function: Copper is important for proper immune function. It is involved in the activation of immune cells and the production of cytokines and antibodies. Copper deficiency can impair immune responses and increase susceptibility to infections.

- Antioxidant Defense: Copper is a component of the antioxidant enzyme superoxide dismutase (SOD), which helps neutralize free radicals and reduce oxidative stress. Copper deficiency can lead to decreased SOD activity and increased oxidative damage to cells and tissues.

Good dietary sources of copper include organ meats (such as liver and kidney), shellfish (such as oysters and crab), nuts and seeds (such as cashews and sesame seeds), legumes, whole grains, dark leafy greens, cocoa, and chocolate. The recommended daily intake of copper varies by age, sex, and life stage, but for most adults, it ranges from 900 to 1300 micrograms per day. While copper deficiency is relatively rare, excessive copper intake can be toxic and lead to adverse health effects, so it's important to consume copper within recommended levels.

Cobalt is a chemical element with atomic number 27 and symbol Co. *Here are some key points about cobalt:*

- Natural Occurrence: Cobalt is a hard, brittle, silver-gray metal that occurs naturally in the Earth's crust. It is primarily obtained as a byproduct of nickel and copper mining, with the largest deposits found in regions such as the Democratic Republic of the Congo, Canada, Australia, and Russia.

- Industrial Uses: Cobalt is widely used in various industrial applications due to its unique properties. It is an important component in the production of alloys, including high-strength steels, super alloys used in aerospace and gas turbine engines, and magnetic materials. Cobalt-based alloys are also used in cutting tools, wear-resistant coatings, and magnets.

- Battery Production: Cobalt is a crucial component in the cathodes of lithium-ion batteries, which are used in rechargeable electronic devices such as smartphones, laptops, and electric vehicles. It helps improve the stability, energy density, and performance of lithium-ion batteries. The growing demand for electric vehicles and renewable energy storage has led to increased demand for cobalt in recent years.

- Health and Medicine: Cobalt has some applications in the field of health and medicine. It is used in the production of vitamin B12, a vital nutrient for human health that plays a role in DNA synthesis, red blood cell formation, and neurological function. Cobalt-based compounds are also used in certain medical implants, such as orthopedic implants and dental prosthetics.

- Radioactive Isotopes: Cobalt has several radioactive isotopes, including cobalt-60, which is used in medical and industrial applications. Cobalt-60 is used in radiation therapy to treat cancer, sterilize medical equipment, and irradiate food to extend shelf life and ensure safety.

- Environmental Concerns: Cobalt mining and processing can have environmental impacts, including habitat destruction, water pollution, and soil contamination. In regions where cobalt mining is prevalent, there have been concerns about labor practices, human rights abuses, and child labor in the cobalt supply chain.

- Safety Precautions: Cobalt and its compounds can be toxic if ingested or inhaled in large amounts. Occupational exposure to cobalt dust or fumes can cause respiratory issues, lung disease, and skin irritation. Proper safety measures should be followed in workplaces where cobalt is handled or processed.

Overall, cobalt plays a significant role in various industries and technologies, but its extraction and use also raise important environmental and social considerations that need to be addressed responsibly.

Manganese is a chemical element with the symbol Mn and atomic number 25. *Here are some key points about manganese:*

- Natural Occurrence: Manganese is a gray-white metal that occurs naturally in the Earth's crust. It is the 12th most abundant element in the Earth's crust and is found in various minerals, rocks, soil, and groundwater. Manganese ores are mined primarily in South Africa, Australia, China, Gabon, and Brazil.

- Industrial Uses: Manganese is widely used in various industrial applications due to its unique properties. It is primarily used as an alloying element in the production of steel and cast iron. Manganese improves the strength, toughness, and hardenability of steel and helps prevent brittleness and cracking during the manufacturing process. Manganese alloys are also used in aluminum alloys, copper alloys, and batteries.

- Battery Production: Manganese is a key component in the production of lithium-ion batteries. Manganese oxide-based cathodes are used in lithium-ion batteries for electric vehicles, portable electronic devices, and energy storage systems. Manganese dioxide is also used in alkaline batteries and dry cell batteries.

- Chemical Compounds: Manganese forms numerous chemical compounds, including oxides, sulfides, halides, and silicates. Manganese dioxide ($MnO2$) is one of the most common manganese compounds and is used in the production of dry cell batteries, water treatment chemicals, and glass manufacturing. Manganese sulfate is used in fertilizers, animal feed supplements, and dietary supplements.

- Health and Nutrition: Manganese is an essential nutrient for human health and is required in small amounts for various physiological functions. It plays a role in bone formation, cartilage formation, wound healing, and metabolism of carbohydrates, proteins, and fats. Manganese is found in a variety of foods, including nuts, seeds, whole grains, legumes, leafy green vegetables, and tea.

- Environmental Concerns: Manganese mining and processing can have environmental impacts, including habitat destruction, water pollution, and soil contamination. Occupational exposure to manganese dust or fumes can pose health risks, including respiratory issues, neurological effects, and toxicity to the nervous system. Proper safety measures should be followed in workplaces where manganese is handled or processed.

- Regulatory Limits: Regulatory agencies, such as the U.S. Environmental Protection Agency (EPA), have established limits for manganese exposure in drinking water and air to protect public health. High levels of manganese in drinking water can cause aesthetic issues (such as discoloration and taste) and potential health risks, particularly for vulnerable populations such as infants and the elderly.

Overall, manganese plays a significant role in various industries and technologies, but its extraction and use also raise important environmental and health considerations that need to be addressed responsibly.

Iodine is a chemical element with the symbol I and atomic number 53. *Here are some key points about iodine:*

- Biological Importance: Iodine is essential for the synthesis of thyroid hormones, which play a crucial role in regulating metabolism, growth, and development. Thyroid hormones, such as thyroxine (T4) and triiodothyronine (T3), contain iodine atoms and are produced by the thyroid gland.

- Thyroid Function: The thyroid gland takes up iodine from the bloodstream and uses it to produce thyroid hormones. Iodine deficiency can lead to thyroid disorders, including hypothyroidism (underactive thyroid) and goiter (enlarged thyroid gland), as the thyroid gland tries to compensate for inadequate iodine levels.

- Dietary Sources: Iodine is found naturally in certain foods and can also be obtained through iodized salt and supplements. Seafood, such as seaweed, fish, and shellfish, is one of the richest dietary sources of iodine. Other sources include dairy products, eggs, and iodized salt.

- Public Health Measures: Iodine deficiency was once a significant public health concern, leading to widespread efforts to fortify salt with iodine (iodized salt) to prevent iodine deficiency disorders. Universal salt iodization programs have been implemented in many countries to ensure adequate iodine intake and prevent iodine-related health problems.

- Pregnancy and Development: Iodine is particularly important during pregnancy and infancy for proper fetal and infant brain development. Severe iodine deficiency during pregnancy can result in congenital hypothyroidism, intellectual disabilities, and other developmental abnormalities in the newborn.

- Thyroid Cancer Treatment: Radioactive iodine (iodine-131) is used in the treatment of thyroid cancer. Radioactive iodine is taken up by thyroid cells, including cancerous cells, and destroys them with radiation. This treatment is known as radioactive iodine therapy and is often used after thyroidectomy (surgical removal of the thyroid gland) to eliminate any remaining thyroid tissue or cancer cells.

- Environmental Impact: Iodine can also be found in the environment in various forms, including iodine-containing compounds in soil and water. Iodine can be released into the atmosphere through natural processes, such as volcanic eruptions, and human activities, such as industrial processes and coal combustion.

Overall, iodine is a vital micronutrient with critical roles in thyroid function, metabolism, and development. Ensuring adequate iodine intake is essential for maintaining overall health and preventing iodine deficiency disorders.

Nickel is a chemical element with the symbol Ni and atomic number 28. *Here are some key points about nickel:*

- Physical Properties: Nickel is a silvery-white metal with a slight golden tinge. It is ductile, meaning it can be stretched into thin wires, and malleable, meaning it can be hammered into thin sheets. Nickel has good corrosion resistance, particularly in alkaline environments, and is highly magnetic.

- Natural Occurrence: Nickel is a relatively abundant element in the Earth's crust, ranking fifth among the transition metals. It is found in various ores and minerals, including pentlandite, pyrrhotite, and garnierite. The largest nickel deposits are located in countries such as Canada, Russia, Australia, and Indonesia.

- Industrial Uses: Nickel is widely used in various industrial applications due to its unique properties. It is primarily used as an alloying element in the production of stainless steel, which accounts for the majority of nickel consumption. Nickel alloys are also used in the aerospace industry, chemical processing equipment, electrical components, and coinage.

- Stainless Steel Production: Nickel is a key component in the production of stainless steel, where it imparts corrosion resistance, strength, and durability to the alloy. Stainless steel is used in a wide range of applications, including construction, architecture, automotive manufacturing, and household appliances.

- Battery Production: Nickel is used in the production of rechargeable batteries, particularly nickel-metal hydride (NiMH) batteries and nickel-cadmium (NiCd) batteries. These batteries are used in various electronic devices, such as mobile phones, laptops, and power tools.

- Health and Safety Concerns: Nickel exposure can have health and safety implications for workers in industries where nickel is mined, processed, or used. Occupational exposure to nickel dust, fumes, or particles can cause respiratory issues, skin allergies, and lung disease. Proper safety measures should be followed in workplaces where nickel is handled or processed to minimize exposure risks.

- Environmental Impact: Nickel mining and processing can have environmental impacts, including habitat destruction, water pollution, and soil contamination. Efforts to mitigate the environmental impact of nickel mining and processing include implementing sustainable practices, reclamation of mined land, and reducing emissions of pollutants.

Overall, nickel plays a significant role in various industries and technologies, but its extraction and use also raise important environmental and health considerations that need to be addressed responsibly.

Fluorine is a chemical element with the symbol F and atomic number 9. *Here are some key points about fluorine:*

- Chemical Properties: Fluorine is the most reactive and electronegative element on the periodic table. It is a pale yellow diatomic gas at room temperature and pressure. Due to its high reactivity, fluorine forms compounds with nearly all other elements.

- Natural Occurrence: Fluorine is relatively rare in nature, occurring primarily in the form of fluoride minerals such as fluorite (calcium fluoride) and fluoroapatite (calcium phosphate). It is also found in trace amounts in rocks, soil, water, and some foods.

- Industrial Uses: Fluorine and its compounds have numerous industrial applications. One of the most significant uses of fluorine is in the production of fluorinated compounds such as hydrofluoric acid, sulfur hexafluoride, and various fluoropolymers. These compounds are used in the manufacture of refrigerants, plastics, textiles, pharmaceuticals, and electronic components.

- Water Fluoridation: Fluoride ions, derived from fluorine compounds such as sodium fluoride or fluorosilicic acid, are added to public water supplies in many countries to prevent tooth decay and promote dental health. Water fluoridation has been shown to be an effective public health measure for reducing dental caries (cavities) in populations.

- Health Considerations: While fluoride is beneficial for dental health when used appropriately, excessive fluoride exposure can lead to dental fluorosis (a cosmetic condition that affects tooth enamel) and skeletal fluorosis (a bone disease caused by excessive fluoride intake). Therefore, it's important to monitor fluoride levels in drinking water and dental products to prevent overexposure.

- Chemical Safety: Fluorine gas is highly toxic and can cause severe burns upon contact with skin or mucous membranes. It reacts violently with water and organic compounds, posing significant safety risks in handling and storage. Special precautions are necessary when working with fluorine or fluorine-containing compounds.

- Environmental Impact: The production and use of fluorine compounds can have environmental impacts, including air and water pollution, as well as the release of greenhouse gases. Efforts to minimize environmental impacts include waste treatment, emission controls, and recycling of fluorine-containing materials.

Overall, fluorine is a highly reactive element with diverse industrial applications and important implications for health and the environment. Proper handling and regulation of fluorine and fluorine-containing compounds are essential to mitigate potential risks and maximize their benefits.

Molybdenum is a chemical element with the symbol Mo and atomic number 42. *Here are some key points about molybdenum*:

- Physical Properties: Molybdenum is a silvery-gray metal with a high melting point of 2,623 degrees Celsius (4,753 degrees Fahrenheit), making it one of the refractory metals. It has a relatively high density and is relatively resistant to corrosion and oxidation at room temperature.

- Natural Occurrence: Molybdenum is a relatively abundant element in the Earth's crust, but it rarely occurs in its pure metallic form. Instead, it is usually found in various minerals, such as molybdenite (a sulfide mineral), wulfenite, and powellite. The largest molybdenum deposits are found in countries such as China, the United States, Chile, and Canada.

- Industrial Uses: Molybdenum has numerous industrial applications due to its unique properties. It is primarily used as an alloying element in the production of high-strength steels, super alloys, and heat-resistant alloys. Molybdenum alloys are used in structural components, tools, aircraft parts, and industrial machinery.

- Catalytic Properties: Molybdenum compounds are used as catalysts in various chemical processes, including petroleum refining, chemical synthesis, and environmental remediation. Molybdenum catalysts are employed in reactions such as hydrodesulphurization (removal of sulfur from petroleum), oxidation, and polymerization.

- Electronics and Electrical Applications: Molybdenum is used in electronics and electrical applications due to its high conductivity and resistance to thermal expansion. It is used in the production of semiconductor devices, electrical contacts, heating elements, and thin-film coatings for integrated circuits.

- Lubrication: Molybdenum disulfide (MoS2) is a solid lubricant that is used in applications where high temperatures, pressures, or extreme environments are present. It reduces friction and wears between moving parts and is used in automotive engines, industrial machinery, and aerospace components.

- Health and Nutrition: Molybdenum is an essential trace element for humans and animals. It is a cofactor for enzymes involved in various metabolic processes, including sulfur metabolism, purine metabolism, and detoxification of certain compounds. Dietary sources of molybdenum include legumes, grains, nuts, leafy vegetables, and meats.

Overall, molybdenum plays a vital role in numerous industrial applications, technological advancements, and biological processes. Its unique properties make it indispensable in various sectors, from manufacturing and engineering to healthcare and nutrition.

Vanadium is a chemical element with the symbol V and atomic number 23. *Here are some key points about vanadium*:

- Physical Properties: Vanadium is a transition metal with a silvery-gray appearance. It is relatively hard, ductile, and malleable. Vanadium has a high melting point of 1,910 degrees Celsius (3,470 degrees Fahrenheit) and is resistant to corrosion.

- Natural Occurrence: Vanadium is found in various minerals, including vanadinite, patronite, and carnotite. It is also present in certain ores, such as titan magnetite and vanadiferous magnetite. Vanadium is primarily mined as a byproduct of other metal ores, such as iron, uranium, and titanium ores.

- Industrial Uses: Vanadium has numerous industrial applications due to its unique properties. It is primarily used as an alloying element in the production of high-strength steels, where it improves strength, toughness, and corrosion resistance. Vanadium alloys are used in structural components, tool steels, and turbine blades.

- Chemical Catalysts: Vanadium compounds are used as catalysts in various chemical processes, including oxidation reactions, polymerization, and sulfuric acid production. Vanadium catalysts are employed in reactions such as the oxidation of sulfur dioxide to sulfur trioxide (used in sulfuric acid manufacture) and the oxidation of alkenes to epoxides.

- Energy Storage: Vanadium redox flow batteries (VRFBs) are a type of rechargeable battery that uses vanadium ions in different oxidation states (vanadium salts) dissolved in a solution as the electrolyte. VRFBs are used for grid-scale energy storage applications due to their high energy efficiency, long cycle life, and scalability.

- Metallurgy: Vanadium is used in metallurgical processes to produce alloys with desirable properties. Vanadium-containing alloys are used in the aerospace industry, where high strength-to-weight ratios and temperature resistance are required. Vanadium alloys are also used in the production of superconducting magnets and high-speed tool steels.

- Biological Role: Vanadium is not considered an essential element for humans, but it has been studied for its potential biological roles. Some organisms, such as certain marine algae and vanadium-dependent nitrogen-fixing bacteria, use vanadium compounds in enzymatic processes. Vanadium compounds have also been investigated for their potential therapeutic effects in treating diabetes and cancer.

Overall, vanadium plays a significant role in various industrial applications, technological advancements, and scientific research. Its unique properties make it indispensable in sectors ranging from metallurgy and energy storage to chemical manufacturing and biomedicine.

Tin is a chemical element with the symbol Sn and atomic number 50. *Here are some key points about tin*:

- Physical Properties: Tin is a soft, silvery-white metal with a relatively low melting point of 231.93 degrees Celsius (449.47 degrees Fahrenheit). It has a high malleability and ductility, making it easy to work with and shape into various forms.

- Natural Occurrence: Tin is relatively abundant in the Earth's crust and is found in various minerals, including cassiterite (tin dioxide), stannite, and teal lite. The largest tin deposits are located in countries such as China, Indonesia, Peru, and Bolivia.
- Historical Uses: Tin has been used by humans for thousands of years. It was one of the earliest metals to be used in the production of bronze, an alloy of copper and tin, which was widely used in ancient civilizations for tools, weapons, and ceremonial objects. Tin was also used to coat other metals to prevent corrosion, a process known as tin plating or tinning.

- Uses Industrial: Tin has numerous industrial applications due to its unique properties. It is primarily used as a coating material for steel and other metals to prevent corrosion and improve solder ability. Tin-plated steel is commonly used in food packaging, beverage cans, and electrical components. Tin alloys, such as bronze and pewter, are used in manufacturing bearings, bearings, and metal parts.

- Soldering: Tin is a key component in solder, a fusible metal alloy used to join or bond metal surfaces together. Soldering is commonly used in electronics assembly, plumbing, and metalwork. Tin-based solders typically contain tin combined with other metals such as lead, silver, or copper.

- Biological Role: Tin is not considered an essential element for humans, and there is limited information on its biological role. However, some tin compounds have been used in medicine as antifungal agents and as food additives, although their use has declined due to concerns about toxicity.

- Environmental Concerns: While tin itself is relatively non-toxic, certain tin compounds can be harmful to human health and the environment. Tin mining and processing can have environmental impacts, including habitat destruction, water pollution, and soil contamination. Efforts to mitigate the environmental impact of tin mining include implementing sustainable practices and responsible mining techniques.

Overall, tin plays a significant role in various industrial applications, historical artifacts, and modern technologies. Its unique properties make it indispensable in sectors ranging from metallurgy and manufacturing to electronics and packaging.

Silicon is a chemical element with the symbol Si and atomic number 14. *Here are some key points about silicon:*

- Abundance: Silicon is the second most abundant element in the Earth's crust, making up about 28% of its mass by weight. It is found in various minerals, rocks, and soils, primarily in the form of silicon dioxide (SiO_2) or silica.

- Physical Properties: Silicon is a metalloid with a grayish appearance and a crystalline structure. It has a relatively high melting point of 1,414 degrees Celsius (2,577 degrees Fahrenheit) and a density lower than that of most metals. Silicon is a poor conductor of electricity in its pure form, but it becomes a semiconductor when doped with impurities.

- Semiconductor Properties: Silicon is widely used in the electronics industry as a semiconductor material. It has unique electrical properties that make it suitable for the production of integrated circuits, transistors, diodes, and other electronic components. Silicon-based semiconductors are the foundation of modern electronics and computing devices.

- Solar Cells: Silicon is used in the production of photovoltaic cells (solar cells) for converting sunlight into electricity. Silicon solar cells are among the most widely used solar cell technologies due to their efficiency, reliability, and relatively low cost. Silicon solar panels are used in residential, commercial, and industrial solar energy systems.

- Silicones: Silicones are synthetic polymers derived from silicon and oxygen atoms, often with organic groups attached. Silicones have a wide range of industrial applications due to their flexibility, heat resistance, water repellency, and biocompatibility. They are used in sealants, adhesives, lubricants, medical implants, and personal care products.

- Metallurgy: Silicon is used as an alloying element in the production of various metals and alloys. Ferrosilicon, an alloy of iron and silicon, is used in steelmaking to improve the strength, hardness, and magnetic properties of steel. Silicon is also used in aluminum alloys to improve their casting properties and mechanical strength.

- Glass and Ceramics: Silicon dioxide (silica) is the primary component of glass and ceramics. Silicon-based glasses and ceramics have high thermal stability, chemical resistance, and optical transparency, making them suitable for a wide range of applications, including windows, lenses, optical fibers, and laboratory equipment.

Overall, silicon plays a crucial role in numerous industrial applications, technological advancements, and everyday products. Its unique properties make it indispensable in sectors ranging from electronics and solar energy to construction and materials science.

Strontium is a chemical element with the symbol Sr and atomic number 38. *Here are some key points about strontium*:

- Physical Properties: Strontium is a soft, silvery-white alkaline earth metal. It is relatively reactive and rapidly oxidizes in air, forming a protective oxide layer on its surface. Strontium has a melting point of 769 degrees Celsius (1,416 degrees Fahrenheit) and a boiling point of 1,384 degrees Celsius (2,523 degrees Fahrenheit).

- Natural Occurrence: Strontium is found naturally in the Earth's crust, primarily in the minerals celestite (strontium sulfate) and strontianite (strontium carbonate). It is also present in small amounts in certain ores, rocks, soil, and groundwater. The largest strontium deposits are located in regions such as the United States, Mexico, Spain, and China.

- Industrial Uses: Strontium has various industrial applications due to its unique properties. One of the most significant uses of strontium compounds is in the production of pyrotechnic materials, such as fireworks and flares. Strontium salts are added to pyrotechnic compositions to produce vivid red colors in flames.

- Medical Applications: Strontium granulate, a strontium salt, has been used in medicine for the treatment of osteoporosis. It is believed to promote bone formation and inhibit bone restoration, helping to increase bone density and reduce the risk of fractures in patients with osteoporosis. However, its use has declined due to safety concerns.

- Nuclear Applications: Strontium-90, a radioactive isotope of strontium, is produced as a byproduct of nuclear fission reactions in nuclear reactors and atomic bomb explosions. Strontium-90 is a major component of radioactive fallout and poses health risks due to its high energy beta radiation. It can accumulate in the bones and cause bone cancer and other health problems.

- Environmental Concerns: Strontium contamination can occur in the environment as a result of industrial activities, mining operations, and nuclear accidents. Strontium-90 released into the atmosphere during nuclear testing and accidents, such as the Chernobyl and Fukushima disasters, can spread over large areas and contaminate soil, water, and food supplies.

- Research and Technology: Strontium has applications in research and technology, including in the field of optics and laser technology. Strontium-based compounds are used in the production of fluorescent pigments, scintillation detectors, and optical glass. Strontium atomic clocks, which use strontium atoms as the timekeeping element, are among the most accurate atomic clocks developed to date.

Overall, while strontium has some industrial and technological applications, its radioactive isotopes and environmental concerns have raised important health and safety considerations. Proper handling and disposal of strontium-containing materials are necessary to minimize potential risks to human health and the environment.

Boron is a chemical element with the symbol B and atomic number 5. *Here are some key points about boron*:

- Physical Properties: Boron is a metalloid with unique physical properties. It exists in several allotropic forms, including amorphous boron, crystalline boron, and boron nanotubes. Crystalline boron is hard and brittle, with a black-brown color.

- Natural Occurrence: Boron is relatively rare in the Earth's crust, typically occurring in compounds rather than in its pure elemental form. Boron compounds are found in various minerals, such as borax, kernite, and colemanite. The largest boron deposits are located in regions such as the United States, Turkey, and Argentina.

- Industrial Uses: Boron has numerous industrial applications due to its unique properties. It is used in the production of borosilicate glass, which has high thermal resistance and chemical durability. Boron compounds are also used in ceramics, detergents, flame retardants, and fiberglass insulation.

- Semiconductor Industry: Boron is used as a dopant in the semiconductor industry to alter the electrical properties of silicon and other semiconductor materials. Boron doping is used to create p-type semiconductor materials, which have excess positive charge carriers (holes).

- Nuclear Applications: Boron-10, a naturally occurring isotope of boron, is used in nuclear reactors as a neutron absorber. Boron-10 absorbs thermal neutrons and undergoes neutron capture, producing alpha particles and lithium-7 nuclei. Boron-10 is also used in neutron detectors and shielding materials.

- Health Benefits: Boron is an essential micronutrient for plants and has been studied for its potential health benefits in humans. Some research suggests that boron may play a role in bone health, cognitive function, and hormone regulation. Boron supplements are sometimes used to support joint health and bone density.

- Environmental Considerations: Boron compounds can have environmental impacts if released into the air, water, or soil. Boron toxicity can occur in plants and animals at high concentrations, leading to stunted growth, reproductive issues, and other health problems. Efforts to minimize boron contamination include proper waste management and pollution control measures.

Overall, boron plays a significant role in various industrial applications, technological advancements, and biological processes. Its unique properties make it indispensable in sectors ranging from glassmaking and ceramics to electronics and agriculture.

VITAMINS

Vitamin A, also known as retinol, is a fat-soluble vitamin that is essential for various physiological functions in the human body. *Here are some key points about vitamin A:*

- Chemical Structure: Vitamin A is a group of unsaturated organic compounds known as retinoid. The most active form of vitamin A in the body is retinol, which can be converted into other biologically active forms such as retinal and retinoic acid.

- Sources: Vitamin A can be obtained from both animal and plant sources. Animal sources of vitamin A include liver, fish liver oil, egg yolks, and dairy products. Plant sources contain provitamin A carotenoids, such as beta-carotene, which can be converted into vitamin A in the body. Rich sources of provitamin A carotenoids include orange and yellow fruits and vegetables, as well as dark leafy greens.

- Functions: Vitamin A plays crucial roles in various physiological processes, including vision, immune function, cell growth and differentiation, reproduction, and skin health. In the eyes, vitamin A is a component of rhodopsin, a pigment that is essential for low-light and color vision. Vitamin A also supports the integrity of mucous membranes, which serve as a barrier against pathogens.

- Vision: Vitamin A is essential for maintaining healthy vision, particularly in low-light conditions. It is involved in the synthesis of visual pigments in the retina, which are necessary for the transduction of light into electrical signals that are transmitted to the brain.

- Immune Function: Vitamin A plays a crucial role in supporting the immune system's response to infections. It helps maintain the integrity of epithelial barriers in the respiratory, gastrointestinal, and genitourinary tracts, which serve as the body's first line of defense against pathogens.

- Cell Growth and Differentiation: Vitamin A is involved in regulating cell growth, differentiation, and apoptosis (programmed cell death). It helps ensure the proper development and function of various tissues and organs, including the skin, bones, and reproductive organs.

- Deficiency: Vitamin A deficiency can lead to a range of health problems, including night blindness, dry eyes, increased susceptibility to infections, impaired growth and development, and reproductive issues. Severe vitamin A deficiency can cause xerophthalmia, a condition characterized by irreversible damage to the cornea and blindness.

- Toxicity: Excessive intake of vitamin A from supplements or animal sources can lead to hypervitaminosis A, which can cause symptoms such as nausea, vomiting, headache, dizziness, and liver damage. Chronic vitamin A toxicity can lead to bone abnormalities, skin changes, and intracranial pressure.

Overall, vitamin A is an essential nutrient that plays critical roles in vision, immune function, growth, and development. Maintaining adequate vitamin A intake through a balanced diet is important for overall health and well-being.

Vitamin B1, also known as thiamine, is a water-soluble vitamin that is essential for various physiological functions in the human body. *Here are some key points about vitamin B1:*

- Chemical Structure: Thiamine is a member of the vitamin B complex and is composed of a diazole ring and a pyrimidine ring linked by a methylene bridge. It is synthesized by plants and microorganisms but must be obtained from the diet by humans.

- Sources: Vitamin B1 is found in a variety of foods, including whole grains, legumes, nuts, seeds, pork, beef, and yeast. Some foods are also fortified with thiamine, such as breakfast cereals and bread.
- Functions: Thiamine plays crucial roles in various metabolic processes, including carbohydrate metabolism, energy production, and nerve function. It serves as a cofactor for several enzymes involved in the conversion of carbohydrates into glucose, which is used as fuel by the body.

- Carbohydrate Metabolism: Thiamine is essential for the breakdown of carbohydrates, particularly glucose, through a series of biochemical reactions known as the Krebs cycle and the pentose phosphate pathway. These pathways generate ATP, the primary energy currency of cells.

- Energy Production: Thiamine is involved in the synthesis of adenosine triphosphate (ATP), a molecule that stores and releases energy in cells. It helps convert the energy obtained from carbohydrates, fats, and proteins into ATP through oxidative phosphorylation in the mitochondria.

- Nerve Function: Thiamine is important for maintaining the health and function of the nervous system. It plays a role in the synthesis of neurotransmitters, such as acetylcholine, which are essential for transmitting nerve impulses. Thiamine deficiency can lead to nerve damage and neurological symptoms.

- Beriberi: Severe thiamine deficiency can lead to a condition known as beriberi, which is characterized by symptoms such as muscle weakness, fatigue, nerve damage, and cardiovascular problems. Beriberi can be classified into two main types: wet beriberi, which affects the cardiovascular system, and dry beriberi, which affects the nervous system.

- Wernicke-Korsakoff Syndrome: Wernicke-Korsakoff syndrome is a neurological disorder caused by severe thiamine deficiency, often associated with chronic alcoholism. It is characterized by symptoms such as confusion, memory loss, ataxia (loss of coordination), and vision changes.

- Recommended Intake: The recommended dietary allowance (RDA) for thiamine varies depending on age, sex, and life stage. For adults, the RDA for thiamine is around 1.2 mg per day for males and 1.1 mg per day for females. Pregnant and lactating women may require higher doses.

Overall, vitamin B1 is an essential nutrient that plays critical roles in carbohydrate metabolism, energy production, and nerve function. Maintaining adequate intake of thiamine through a balanced diet is important for overall health and well-being.

Vitamin B2, also known as riboflavin, is a water-soluble vitamin that is essential for various physiological functions in the human body. *Here are some key points about vitamin B2:*

- Chemical Structure: Riboflavin is a member of the vitamin B complex and is composed of a central isoalloxazine ring system with a ribityl side chain. It is synthesized by plants, bacteria, and fungi but must be obtained from the diet by humans.
- Sources: Vitamin B2 is found in a variety of foods, including dairy products (such as milk, yogurt, and cheese), eggs, meat (such as liver and poultry), fish, green leafy vegetables, whole grains, and fortified cereals.

- Functions: Riboflavin plays crucial roles in various metabolic processes, including energy production, antioxidant defense, and red blood cell formation. It serves as a precursor for two coenzymes: flavin mononucleotide (FMN) and flavin adenine dinucleotide (FAD), which are involved in numerous enzymatic reactions.

- Energy Production: Riboflavin is essential for the metabolism of carbohydrates, fats, and proteins. As a component of FMN and FAD, it acts as a cofactor for enzymes involved in oxidative phosphorylation, the process by which cells generate adenosine triphosphate (ATP), the primary energy currency of cells.

- Antioxidant Defense: Riboflavin, in its active coenzyme forms (FMN and FAD), participates in antioxidant reactions that help protect cells from oxidative damage caused by free radicals and reactive oxygen species. It helps regenerate other antioxidants, such as glutathione and vitamin E, and supports the function of antioxidant enzymes.

- Red Blood Cell Formation: Riboflavin is involved in the synthesis of red blood cells (erythrocytes) and the maintenance of normal hemoglobin levels. It plays a role in the production of heme, the iron-containing component of hemoglobin, which is responsible for transporting oxygen in the blood.

- Skin and Eye Health: Riboflavin is important for maintaining the health of the skin, eyes, and mucous membranes. It contributes to the production of collagen, a protein that provides structural support to the skin and other tissues. Riboflavin deficiency can lead to skin disorders, such as dermatitis, and eye conditions, such as photophobia (sensitivity to light) and blurred vision.

- Recommended Intake: The recommended dietary allowance (RDA) for riboflavin varies depending on age, sex, and life stage. For adults, the RDA for riboflavin is around 1.3 mg per day for males and 1.1 mg per day for females. Pregnant and lactating women may require higher doses.

Overall, vitamin B2 is an essential nutrient that plays critical roles in energy metabolism, antioxidant defense, red blood cell formation, and skin and eye health. Maintaining adequate intake of riboflavin through a balanced diet is important for overall health and well-being.

Vitamin B3, also known as niacin or nicotinic acid, is a water-soluble vitamin that is essential for various physiological functions in the human body. *Here are some key points about vitamin B3:*

- Chemical Structure: Niacin is a member of the vitamin B complex and exists in several forms, including nicotinic acid (niacin), nicotinamide (niacinamide), and nicotinamide riboside. It is synthesized in the body from the amino acid tryptophan, but dietary sources of niacin are also important.

- Sources: Vitamin B3 is found in a variety of foods, including meat (such as poultry, fish, and beef liver), poultry, fish, whole grains (such as wheat, barley, and oats), legumes (such as peanuts and lentils), nuts, seeds, and fortified cereals.

- Functions: Niacin plays crucial roles in various metabolic processes, including energy production, DNA repair, and synthesis of certain hormones and neurotransmitters. It serves as a precursor for two coenzymes: nicotinamide adenine dinucleotide (NAD) and nicotinamide adenine dinucleotide phosphate (NADP), which are involved in numerous enzymatic reactions.

- Energy Production: Niacin is essential for the metabolism of carbohydrates, fats, and proteins. As a component of NAD and NADP, it acts as a cofactor for enzymes involved in oxidative phosphorylation, the process by which cells generate adenosine triphosphate (ATP), the primary energy currency of cells.

- DNA Repair: Niacin plays a role in DNA repair mechanisms, helping to maintain the integrity of the genetic material and prevent mutations and DNA damage. It contributes to the synthesis of poly (ADP-ribose) polymerase (PARP), an enzyme involved in DNA repair processes.

- Hormone and Neurotransmitter Synthesis: Niacin is involved in the synthesis of certain hormones and neurotransmitters, including adrenal hormones (such as cortisol), sex hormones (such as estrogen and testosterone), and neurotransmitters (such as serotonin). It contributes to the production of tryptophan hydroxylase, an enzyme involved in serotonin synthesis.

- Cholesterol and Lipid Metabolism: Niacin has been shown to have lipid-lowering effects, particularly on low-density lipoprotein (LDL) cholesterol and triglycerides, while increasing high-density lipoprotein (HDL) cholesterol levels. It works by inhibiting the synthesis of cholesterol and triglycerides in the liver and promoting their clearance from the bloodstream.

- Pellagra: Severe niacin deficiency can lead to a condition known as pellagra, which is characterized by symptoms such as dermatitis (skin rash), diarrhea, dementia, and death if left untreated. Pellagra was historically common in populations whose diets were deficient in niacin-rich foods, such as maize-based diets.
- Recommended Intake: The recommended dietary allowance (RDA) for niacin varies depending on age, sex, and life stage. For adults, the RDA for niacin is around 16 mg per day for males and 14 mg per day for females. Pregnant and lactating women may require higher doses.

Overall, vitamin B3 is an essential nutrient that plays critical roles in energy metabolism, DNA repair, hormone and neurotransmitter synthesis, and lipid metabolism. Maintaining adequate intake of niacin through a balanced diet is important for overall health and well-being.

Vitamin B6, also known as pyridoxine, is a water-soluble vitamin that is essential for various physiological functions in the human body. *Here are some key points about vitamin B6:*

- Chemical Structure: Pyridoxine is a member of the vitamin B complex and exists in several related forms, including pyridoxine, pyridoxal, pyridoxamine, and their phosphorylated derivatives. These forms can be interconverted in the body.

- Sources: Vitamin B6 is found in a variety of foods, including poultry, fish, meat (such as beef and pork), eggs, nuts, seeds, whole grains, legumes, fruits, and vegetables (such as potatoes and spinach). Fortified cereals and supplements are also sources of vitamin B6.

- Functions: Vitamin B6 plays crucial roles in various metabolic processes, including amino acid metabolism, neurotransmitter synthesis, hemoglobin synthesis, and immune function. It serves as a cofactor for over 100 enzymes involved in these processes.

- Amino Acid Metabolism: Vitamin B6 is involved in the metabolism of amino acids, the building blocks of proteins. It participates in the conversion of amino acids into other compounds, such as neurotransmitters, hormones, and energy sources. Pyridoxal phosphate (PLP), the active form of vitamin B6, acts as a cofactor for enzymes involved in these reactions.

- Neurotransmitter Synthesis: Vitamin B6 is essential for the synthesis of neurotransmitters, such as serotonin, dopamine, and gamma-amino butyric acid (GABA). These neurotransmitters play crucial roles in mood regulation, cognitive function, and sleep-wake cycles. Vitamin B6 deficiency can lead to neurological symptoms due to impaired neurotransmitter synthesis.

- Hemoglobin Synthesis: Vitamin B6 is involved in the synthesis of hemoglobin, the protein in red blood cells that carries oxygen from the lungs to the tissues. It helps convert the amino acid tryptophan into niacin (vitamin B3), which is a precursor for hemoglobin synthesis. Vitamin B6 deficiency can lead to anemia due to impaired hemoglobin production.

- Immune Function: Vitamin B6 plays a role in immune function by supporting the production and function of white blood cells, which are involved in the body's defense against pathogens and foreign invaders. It helps regulate the production of cytokines and other immune signaling molecules.

- Pregnancy and Fetal Development: Vitamin B6 is important for pregnant women and fetal development. It is involved in the synthesis of neurotransmitters and other molecules crucial for brain development. Adequate intake of vitamin B6 during pregnancy is important for preventing birth defects and supporting healthy fetal growth.

- Recommended Intake: The recommended dietary allowance (RDA) for vitamin B6 varies depending on age, sex, and life stage. For adults, the RDA for vitamin B6 is around 1.3-1.7 mg per day. Pregnant and lactating women may require higher doses.

Overall, vitamin B6 is an essential nutrient that plays critical roles in amino acid metabolism, neurotransmitter synthesis, hemoglobin synthesis, immune function, and fetal development. Maintaining adequate intake of vitamin B6 through a balanced diet is important for overall health and well-being.

Vitamin B12, also known as cobalamin, is a water-soluble vitamin that is essential for various physiological functions in the human body. *Here are some key points about vitamin B12:*

- Chemical Structure: Vitamin B12 is a complex molecule that contains cobalt at its center. It exists in several forms, including cyanocobalamin, hydroxocobalamin, methylcobalamin, and adenosylcobalamin. Methylcobalamin and adenosylcobalamin are the active forms of vitamin B12 in the body.

- Sources: Vitamin B12 is found primarily in animal-derived foods, including meat (such as beef, poultry, and fish), dairy products (such as milk, cheese, and yogurt), eggs, and shellfish. Plant-based sources of vitamin B12 are limited, but some fortified foods (such as breakfast cereals, plant-based milk alternatives, and nutritional yeast) contain synthetic vitamin B12.

- Functions: Vitamin B12 plays crucial roles in various metabolic processes, including DNA synthesis, red blood cell formation, nerve function, and homocysteine metabolism. It serves as a cofactor for enzymes involved in these processes.

- DNA Synthesis: Vitamin B12 is essential for the synthesis of DNA, the genetic material found in cells. It is involved in the conversion of homocysteine to methionine, an amino acid that is required for DNA synthesis and cell division.

Red Blood Cell Formation: Vitamin B12 is necessary for the production of red blood cells (erythrocytes) in the bone marrow. It works in conjunction with folate (vitamin B9) to regulate the synthesis of hemoglobin, the protein in red blood cells that carries oxygen from the lungs to the tissues.

- Nerve Function: Vitamin B12 plays a crucial role in maintaining the health and function of the nervous system. It is involved in the synthesis of myelin, a fatty substance that forms a protective sheath around nerves and facilitates the transmission of nerve impulses. Vitamin B12 deficiency can lead to neurological symptoms, such as tingling or numbness in the hands and feet, difficulty walking, and cognitive impairment.

- Homocysteine Metabolism: Vitamin B12, along with folate and vitamin B6, helps regulate the metabolism of homocysteine, an amino acid that can accumulate in the blood if not properly metabolized. Elevated levels of homocysteine are associated with an increased risk of cardiovascular disease, so adequate intake of vitamin B12 is important for heart health.

- Pernicious Anemia: Severe vitamin B12 deficiency can lead to a condition known as pernicious anemia, which is characterized by a lack of intrinsic factor, a protein produced by the stomach that is necessary for vitamin B12 absorption. Pernicious anemia can result in symptoms such as fatigue, weakness, shortness of breath, and pale skin.

- Recommended Intake: The recommended dietary allowance (RDA) for vitamin B12 varies depending on age, sex, and life stage. For adults, the RDA for vitamin B12 is around 2.4 micrograms per day. Pregnant and lactating women may require higher doses.

Overall, vitamin B12 is an essential nutrient that plays critical roles in DNA synthesis, red blood cell formation, nerve function, and homocysteine metabolism. Maintaining adequate intake of vitamin B12 through a balanced diet is important for overall health and well-being.

Vitamin C, also known as ascorbic acid, is a water-soluble vitamin that is essential for various physiological functions in the human body. *Here are some key points about vitamin C:*

- Chemical Structure: Vitamin C is a six-carbon compound with the chemical formula $C_6H_8O_6$. It is a white, crystalline substance that is easily soluble in water. Unlike most animals, humans are unable to synthesize vitamin C endogenously and must obtain it from the diet.

- Sources: Vitamin C is found in a variety of fruits and vegetables, particularly citrus fruits (such as oranges, lemons, and grapefruits), berries (such as strawberries, raspberries, and blueberries), kiwifruit, tomatoes, bell peppers (particularly red peppers), broccoli, Brussels sprouts, and leafy greens (such as kale and spinach).

- Functions: Vitamin C plays crucial roles in various physiological processes, including collagen synthesis, antioxidant defense, immune function, wound healing, and iron absorption. It serves as a cofactor for enzymes involved in these processes.

- Collagen Synthesis: Vitamin C is essential for the synthesis of collagen, a protein that provides structural support to tissues such as skin, bones, cartilage, and blood vessels. It is involved in the hydroxylation of proline and lysine residues in collagen precursors, which is necessary for the formation of stable collagen fibers.

- Antioxidant Defense: Vitamin C is a powerful antioxidant that helps protect cells from damage caused by free radicals and reactive oxygen species. It scavenges free radicals and regenerates other antioxidants, such as vitamin E, glutathione, and coenzyme Q10, enhancing the body's antioxidant defense system.

- Immune Function: Vitamin C plays a role in supporting the immune system's response to infections and inflammation. It helps stimulate the production and function of white blood cells, such as neutrophils, lymphocytes, and phagocytes, which are involved in the body's defense against pathogens.

- Wound Healing: Vitamin C is important for wound healing and tissue repair processes. It promotes the synthesis of collagen and other extracellular matrix components, enhances fibroblast proliferation and migration, and supports angiogenesis (the formation of new blood vessels), which are essential for the healing of wounds.

- Iron Absorption: Vitamin C enhances the absorption of non-heme iron (the form of iron found in plant-based foods and iron supplements) by reducing ferric iron (Fe^{3+}) to ferrous iron (Fe^{2+}), which is more readily absorbed in the intestine. Consuming vitamin C-rich foods or supplements with iron-containing meals can help improve iron absorption, particularly for individuals at risk of iron deficiency.

- Recommended Intake: The recommended dietary allowance (RDA) for vitamin C varies depending on age, sex, and life stage. For adults, the RDA for vitamin C is around 75-90 milligrams per day for males and females. Pregnant and lactating women may require higher doses.

Overall, vitamin C is an essential nutrient that plays critical roles in collagen synthesis, antioxidant defense, immune function, wound healing, and iron absorption. Maintaining adequate intake of vitamin C through a balanced diet rich in fruits and vegetables is important for overall health and well-being.

Vitamin D3, also known as cholecalciferol, is a fat-soluble vitamin that is essential for various physiological functions in the human body. *Here are some key points about vitamin D3:*

- Chemical Structure: Vitamin D3 is a steroid hormone precursor and is derived from cholesterol. It is produced in the skin when exposed to ultraviolet B (UVB) radiation from sunlight. Vitamin D3 can also be obtained from dietary sources or supplements.

- Sources: Vitamin D3 is found in limited amounts in certain foods, including fatty fish (such as salmon, mackerel, and tuna), fish liver oils, egg yolks, and fortified foods (such as milk, orange juice, and breakfast cereals). However, the primary source of vitamin D3 for most people is sunlight exposure.

- Sunlight Exposure: The body can synthesize vitamin D3 in the skin when exposed to UVB radiation from sunlight. Ultraviolet (UV) rays penetrate the skin and convert 7-dehydrocholesterol, a precursor molecule present in the skin, into pre vitamin D3, which is then rapidly converted into vitamin D3. Factors such as time of day, season, latitude, skin pigmentation, and sunscreen use can affect vitamin D3 synthesis.

- Functions: Vitamin D3 plays crucial roles in various physiological processes, including calcium and phosphorus metabolism, bone health, immune function, and cell growth and differentiation. It acts as a hormone that regulates gene expression in target tissues throughout the body.

- Calcium and Phosphorus Metabolism: Vitamin D3 promotes the absorption of calcium and phosphorus from the intestines into the bloodstream and regulates their levels in the blood. It helps maintain calcium homeostasis and supports the mineralization of bones and teeth.

- Bone Health: Vitamin D3 is essential for bone health and the prevention of conditions such as rickets in children and osteomalacia in adults. It facilitates the absorption of calcium and phosphorus by osteoblasts (bone-forming cells) and regulates the activity of osteoclasts (bone-resorbing cells), contributing to bone mineralization and remodeling.

- Immune Function: Vitamin D3 plays a role in modulating the immune system and promoting immune function. It helps regulate the production and activity of immune cells, such as T cells, B cells, and macrophages, and the secretion of cytokines and other immune signaling molecules.

- Cell Growth and Differentiation: Vitamin D3 is involved in regulating cell growth, proliferation, and differentiation in various tissues and organs, including the skin, prostate, breast, colon, and immune system. It helps maintain tissue homeostasis and may have implications for cancer prevention and treatment.

- Recommended Intake: The recommended dietary allowance (RDA) for vitamin D varies depending on age, sex, and life stage. For adults, the RDA for vitamin D is around 600-800 international units (IU) per day. However, individual requirements may vary based on factors such as sunlight exposure, skin pigmentation, and underlying health conditions.

Overall, vitamin D3 is an essential nutrient that plays critical roles in calcium and phosphorus metabolism, bone health, immune function, and cell growth and differentiation. Maintaining adequate intake of vitamin D3 through a combination of sunlight exposure, dietary sources, and supplements is important for overall health and well-being.

Vitamin E is a fat-soluble vitamin that acts as an antioxidant in the body, helping to protect cells from damage caused by free radicals and reactive oxygen species. *Here are some key points about vitamin E:*

- Chemical Structure: Vitamin E refers to a group of compounds known as tocopherols and tocotrienols. The most biologically active form of vitamin E is alpha-tocopherol, although other forms such as beta-, gamma-, and delta-tocopherol also contribute to its antioxidant activity.

- Sources: Vitamin E is found in a variety of foods, particularly plant-based oils (such as wheat germ oil, sunflower oil, safflower oil, and olive oil), nuts and seeds (such as almonds, peanuts, sunflower seeds, and hazelnuts), green leafy vegetables (such as spinach and kale), and fortified foods (such as cereals and spreads).

- Functions: Vitamin E acts primarily as an antioxidant, neutralizing free radicals and reactive oxygen species generated during normal cellular metabolism and in response to environmental stressors such as UV radiation and pollution. It helps protect cell membranes, lipids, proteins, and DNA from oxidative damage.

- Antioxidant Activity: Vitamin E's antioxidant activity is thought to play a role in reducing the risk of chronic diseases such as cardiovascular disease, cancer, and age-related macular degeneration. It helps maintain the integrity and function of cell membranes, which is particularly important for cells exposed to high levels of oxidative stress, such as red blood cells and immune cells.
- Immune Function: Vitamin E may have immune modulatory effects, influencing the function of various components of the immune system. It helps regulate the production and activity of immune cells, such as T cells, B cells, natural killer cells, and macrophages, as well as the secretion of cytokines and other immune signaling molecules.

- Skin Health: Vitamin E is often included in skincare products due to its potential benefits for skin health. It has moisturizing properties and may help protect the skin from damage caused by UV radiation and environmental pollutants. Vitamin E is also thought to have anti-inflammatory effects, which may help reduce skin redness and irritation.

- Heart Health: Some research suggests that vitamin E supplementation may have cardiovascular benefits, such as reducing the risk of coronary heart disease and improving endothelial function. However, the evidence is mixed, and more research is needed to clarify the role of vitamin E in heart health.

- Recommended Intake: The recommended dietary allowance (RDA) for vitamin E varies depending on age, sex, and life stage. For adults, the RDA for vitamin E is around 15 milligrams of alpha-tocopherol equivalents (mg alpha-TE) per day. Pregnant and lactating women may require slightly higher doses.

Overall, vitamin E is an essential nutrient with potent antioxidant properties that help protect cells and tissues from oxidative damage. Maintaining adequate intake of vitamin E through a balanced diet rich in fruits, vegetables, nuts, seeds, and plant-based oils is important for overall health and well-being.

Vitamin K is a fat-soluble vitamin that is essential for blood clotting and bone health. *Here are some key points about vitamin K:*

- Chemical Structure: Vitamin K refers to a group of compounds known as quinines, with two main forms: vitamin K1 (phylloquinone) and vitamin K2 (menaquinone). Vitamin K1 is found primarily in green leafy vegetables, while vitamin K2 is found in animal products and fermented foods.

- Sources: Vitamin K1 is found in green leafy vegetables (such as spinach, kale, broccoli, and Swiss chard), as well as vegetable oils (such as soybean oil and canola oil). Vitamin K2 is found in meat, cheese, eggs, and fermented foods (such as natto, a Japanese soybean dish).

- Functions: Vitamin K is primarily known for its role in blood clotting, where it helps activate proteins involved in the coagulation cascade. These proteins, including prothrombin and factors VII, IX, and X, require vitamin K-dependent gamma-carboxylation for their activation. Vitamin K also plays a role in bone metabolism, where it helps regulate calcium deposition in bone tissue.

- Blood Clotting: Vitamin K is essential for the synthesis of clotting factors in the liver, which are necessary for the formation of blood clots in response to injury or bleeding. Without adequate vitamin K, blood clotting may be impaired, leading to an increased risk of bleeding and hemorrhage.

- Bone Health: Vitamin K is involved in the regulation of bone metabolism and mineralization. It helps activate osteocalcin, a protein that binds calcium ions and facilitates their incorporation into bone tissue. Vitamin K also helps inhibit the activity of osteoclasts, cells that break down bone tissue, thereby supporting bone density and strength.

- Cardiovascular Health: Some research suggests that vitamin K may have cardiovascular benefits, such as reducing the risk of arterial calcification and cardiovascular disease. Vitamin K-dependent proteins, such as matrix Gla protein (MGP), help inhibit the calcification of arterial walls and may have protective effects on the cardiovascular system.

- Recommended Intake: The recommended dietary allowance (RDA) for vitamin K varies depending on age, sex, and life stage. For adults, the Adequate Intake (AI) for vitamin K is around 90-120 micrograms per day for males and 90-110 micrograms per day for females. Pregnant and lactating women may require slightly higher doses.

- Deficiency: Vitamin K deficiency is rare in healthy individuals but can occur in certain populations, such as newborns (due to insufficient vitamin K transfer from the mother and limited vitamin K synthesis by gut bacteria), people with malabsorption disorders (such as celiac disease or inflammatory bowel disease), and those taking medications that interfere with vitamin K metabolism (such as certain anticoagulants).

Overall, vitamin K is an essential nutrient that plays critical roles in blood clotting and bone health. Maintaining adequate intake of vitamin K through a balanced diet rich in green leafy vegetables, vegetable oils, meat, and fermented foods is important for overall health and well-being.

AMINO ACID

Lysine is an essential amino acid, meaning that the body cannot produce it on its own and it must be obtained from the diet. *Here are some key points about lysine:*

- Amino Acid Structure: Lysine is one of the twenty amino acids that are the building blocks of proteins. It has a basic, positively charged amino group (NH_2) at one end, which makes it a basic amino acid, and a carboxyl group ($COOH$) at the other end.

- Role in Protein Synthesis: Lysine plays a crucial role in protein synthesis, where it is incorporated into proteins according to the genetic code. It is particularly important for the formation of collagen, the structural protein found in connective tissues such as skin, tendons, and bones.

- Collagen Formation: Lysine is essential for the synthesis of collagen, where it contributes to the stability and structure of collagen molecules. Lysine residues in collagen molecules form cross-links with other amino acids, such as hydroxyproline and hydroxylysine, to create a strong and flexible collagen matrix.

- Connective Tissue Health: Lysine is important for maintaining the health and integrity of connective tissues throughout the body. It supports the formation of collagen and other extracellular matrix components, which provide structural support and elasticity to tissues such as skin, cartilage, and blood vessels.

- Bone Health: Lysine may play a role in promoting bone health by supporting collagen synthesis and mineralization. Collagen provides the framework for bone tissue, while lysine residues in collagen molecules help bind calcium ions and facilitate their incorporation into bone mineral crystals.

- Immune Function: Lysine may have immunomodulatory effects and contribute to immune function. It is involved in the production of antibodies, enzymes, and other immune system components, and may help support the body's defense against infections and diseases.

- Dietary Sources: Lysine is found in a variety of protein-rich foods, including meat (such as beef, poultry, pork, and fish), dairy products (such as milk, cheese, and yogurt), eggs, soy products (such as tofu and tempeh), legumes (such as beans, lentils, and peas), nuts, seeds, and quinoa.

- Supplementation: Lysine supplements are sometimes used to treat or prevent certain conditions, such as herpes simplex virus infections (cold sores) and herpes zoster (shingles). Lysine supplementation may help reduce the frequency, severity, and duration of herpes outbreaks by interfering with the replication of the virus.

Overall, lysine is an essential amino acid that plays critical roles in protein synthesis, collagen formation, connective tissue health, bone health, and immune function. Maintaining adequate intake of lysine through a balanced diet rich in protein sources is important for overall health and well-being.

Tryptophan is an essential amino acid, meaning that the body cannot produce it and it must be obtained from the diet. *Here are some key points about tryptophan:*

- Amino Acid Structure: Tryptophan is one of the twenty amino acids that are the building blocks of proteins. It has a chemical structure consisting of an indole ring, making it unique among the amino acids. Tryptophan contains an amino group (NH2) and a carboxyl group (COOH), along with a side chain containing the indole ring.

- Role in Protein Synthesis: Tryptophan plays a crucial role in protein synthesis, where it is incorporated into proteins according to the genetic code. It is involved in the formation of peptide bonds that link amino acids together to form polypeptide chains, which ultimately fold into functional proteins.

- Precursor to Neurotransmitters: Tryptophan serves as a precursor for the synthesis of several important neurotransmitters in the brain, including serotonin and melatonin. Serotonin is a neurotransmitter involved in regulating mood, appetite, sleep, and other physiological processes, while melatonin regulates the sleep-wake cycle and circadian rhythms.

- Serotonin Synthesis: Tryptophan is the precursor for serotonin synthesis in the brain. It is converted into 5-hydroxytryptophan (5-HTP) by the enzyme tryptophan hydroxylase, and then further metabolized into serotonin by the enzyme aromatic L-amino acid decarboxylase. Serotonin levels in the brain are influenced by dietary tryptophan intake, as well as factors such as insulin secretion and competition with other amino acids for transport across the blood-brain barrier.

- Mood Regulation: Tryptophan and serotonin are closely linked to mood regulation and emotional well-being. Adequate levels of serotonin in the brain are associated with positive mood, while serotonin deficiency is linked to mood disorders such as depression and anxiety. Increasing dietary tryptophan intake or supplementing with tryptophan may help support serotonin production and improve mood in some individuals.

- Sleep Regulation: Tryptophan is also a precursor for the synthesis of melatonin, a hormone that regulates the sleep-wake cycle and promotes sleep onset. Melatonin levels in the brain rise in response to darkness and decline in response to light, helping to synchronize the body's internal clock with the day-night cycle. Increasing dietary tryptophan intake may help enhance melatonin production and improve sleep quality.

- Dietary Sources: Tryptophan is found in a variety of protein-rich foods, particularly animal-based sources such as poultry (such as turkey and chicken), meat (such as beef and pork), fish, eggs, and dairy products (such as milk, cheese, and yogurt). Plant-based sources of tryptophan include legumes (such as beans, lentils, and peas), nuts, seeds, and whole grains (such as oats and wheat).

- Supplementation: Tryptophan supplements are sometimes used to treat or prevent certain conditions, such as depression, anxiety, insomnia, and seasonal affective disorder (SAD). However, the effectiveness of tryptophan supplementation for these purposes may vary, and it is important to consult with a healthcare professional before starting any supplementation regimen.

Overall, tryptophan is an essential amino acid that plays critical roles in protein synthesis, neurotransmitter synthesis, mood regulation, and sleep regulation. Maintaining adequate intake of tryptophan through a balanced diet rich in protein sources is important for overall health and well-being, particularly for supporting mental health and emotional well-being.

Phenylalanine is an essential amino acid, meaning that it cannot be synthesized by the body and must be obtained from the diet. *Here are some key points about phenylalanine:*

- Amino Acid Structure: Phenylalanine is one of the twenty amino acids that are the building blocks of proteins. It is an aromatic amino acid with a phenyl group as its side chain. There are three forms of phenylalanine: L-phenylalanine, D-phenylalanine, and DL-phenylalanine. The L-form is the biologically active form and is the one found in proteins.

- Role in Protein Synthesis: Phenylalanine is incorporated into proteins during protein synthesis according to the genetic code. It participates in peptide bond formation, linking amino acids together to form polypeptide chains, which ultimately fold into functional proteins.

- Precursor to Neurotransmitters: Phenylalanine is a precursor for the synthesis of several important neurotransmitters in the brain, including dopamine, norepinephrine, and epinephrine. These neurotransmitters play key roles in regulating mood, motivation, attention, and stress response.

- Phenylketonuria (PKU): Phenylalanine metabolism is disrupted in individuals with phenylketonuria (PKU), a rare genetic disorder caused by a deficiency of the enzyme phenylalanine hydroxylase, which is responsible for converting phenylalanine into tyrosine. Without this enzyme, phenylalanine levels in the blood can become elevated, leading to neurological complications and intellectual disabilities. Individuals with PKU must follow a strict low-phenylalanine diet and may require medical treatment to manage their condition.

- Dietary Sources: Phenylalanine is found in a variety of protein-rich foods, particularly animal-based sources such as meat (such as beef, pork, and poultry), fish, eggs, dairy products (such as milk, cheese, and yogurt), and some plant-based sources such as soy products (such as tofu and tempeh), nuts, seeds, and legumes (such as beans and lentils).

- Aspartame: Phenylalanine is a component of the artificial sweetener aspartame, which is used as a sugar substitute in many diet and low-calorie food and beverage products. Individuals with PKU must avoid products containing aspartame, as it can contribute to elevated phenylalanine levels in the blood.

- Phenylalanine Supplementation: Phenylalanine supplements are sometimes used for certain purposes, such as to support mood and cognitive function or to alleviate chronic pain. D-phenylalanine supplements are sometimes used to relieve pain by inhibiting the breakdown of endorphins and encephalin, natural pain-relieving substances in the body.

Overall, phenylalanine is an essential amino acid that plays critical roles in protein synthesis, neurotransmitter synthesis, and overall health. Maintaining adequate intake of phenylalanine through a balanced diet rich in protein sources is important for supporting various physiological functions in the body. However, individuals with PKU must closely monitor their phenylalanine intake to prevent complications associated with elevated blood phenylalanine levels.

Methionine is an essential amino acid, meaning that it cannot be synthesized by the body and must be obtained from the diet. *Here are some key points about methionine:*

- Amino Acid Structure: Methionine is one of the twenty amino acids that are the building blocks of proteins. It has a sulfur-containing side chain and is classified as a sulfur-containing amino acid. The chemical structure of methionine includes an amino group (NH2), a carboxyl group (COOH), and a side chain containing a sulfur atom.

- Role in Protein Synthesis: Methionine plays a crucial role in protein synthesis, where it is incorporated into proteins according to the genetic code. It serves as the "initiator" amino acid for protein translation, meaning that it is the first amino acid added to the growing polypeptide chain during protein synthesis.

- Sulfur Source: Methionine is a major dietary source of sulfur, an essential element for various physiological processes in the body. Sulfur is a component of sulfur-containing amino acids, such as methionine and cysteine, as well as other sulfur-containing compounds involved in metabolism, antioxidant defense, and detoxification.

- Methylation Reactions: Methionine is involved in methylation reactions, where it donates a methyl group (-CH3) to other molecules to facilitate various biochemical processes. Methylation reactions are important for the regulation of gene expression, protein function, neurotransmitter synthesis, and many other cellular processes.

- Antioxidant Defense: Methionine contributes to antioxidant defense mechanisms in the body by serving as a precursor for the synthesis of glutathione, a major antioxidant molecule. Glutathione helps neutralize free radicals and reactive oxygen species, protecting cells and tissues from oxidative damage.

- Detoxification: Methionine is involved in the synthesis of glutathione, which plays a key role in detoxification processes in the liver and other tissues. Glutathione acts as a cofactor for enzymes involved in the metabolism and elimination of toxins, heavy metals, and other harmful substances from the body.

- Dietary Sources: Methionine is found in a variety of protein-rich foods, particularly animal-based sources such as meat (such as beef, poultry, pork, and fish), eggs, dairy products (such as milk, cheese, and yogurt), and some plant-based sources such as soy products (such as tofu and tempeh), nuts, seeds, and legumes (such as beans and lentils).

- Supplementation: Methionine supplements are sometimes used for certain purposes, such as to support liver health, detoxification, and athletic performance. However, excessive methionine intake from supplements may have adverse effects and should be used with caution.

Overall, methionine is an essential amino acid that plays critical roles in protein synthesis, sulfur metabolism, methylation reactions, antioxidant defense, and detoxification. Maintaining adequate intake of methionine through a balanced diet rich in protein sources is important for overall health and well-being.

Threonine is an essential amino acid, meaning that it cannot be synthesized by the body and must be obtained from the diet. *Here are some key points about threonine:*

- Amino Acid Structure: Threonine is one of the twenty amino acids that are the building blocks of proteins. It is classified as a polar, uncharged amino acid and contains a hydroxyl group (-OH) in its side chain. The chemical structure of threonine includes an amino group (NH2), a carboxyl group (COOH), and a side chain containing the hydroxyl group.

- Role in Protein Synthesis: Threonine plays a crucial role in protein synthesis, where it is incorporated into proteins according to the genetic code. It participates in peptide bond formation, linking amino acids together to form polypeptide chains, which ultimately fold into functional proteins.

- Post-translational Modifications: Threonine residues in proteins can undergo various post-translational modifications, including phosphorylation, glycosylation, and hydroxylation. These modifications can alter the structure, function, and stability of proteins, as well as regulate cellular processes such as signal transduction, gene expression, and protein trafficking.

- Glycine and Serine Biosynthesis: Threonine is a precursor for the biosynthesis of other amino acids, including glycine and serine. In a series of enzymatic reactions, threonine is converted into glycine via the intermediate 2-oxobutanoate, and into serine via the intermediate 2-oxopropanoate. Glycine and serine are important for various physiological processes, including protein synthesis, neurotransmitter synthesis, and one-carbon metabolism.

- Mucin Production: Threonine is involved in the synthesis of mucin proteins, which are major components of mucus secretions in the body. Mucins provide lubrication and protection to epithelial surfaces, such as the gastrointestinal tract, respiratory tract, and reproductive tract, and play a role in innate immunity and host defense against pathogens.

- Collagen and Elastin Formation: Threonine is important for the synthesis of structural proteins such as collagen and elastin, which are essential for the integrity and elasticity of connective tissues such as skin, tendons, ligaments, and blood vessels. Threonine residues in collagen molecules contribute to the stability and structure of collagen fibers.

- Dietary Sources: Threonine is found in a variety of protein-rich foods, particularly animal-based sources such as meat (such as beef, poultry, pork, and fish), eggs, dairy products (such as milk, cheese, and yogurt), and some plant-based sources such as soy products (such as tofu and tempeh), nuts, seeds, and legumes (such as beans and lentils).

- Supplementation: Threonine supplements are generally not necessary for most individuals, as adequate amounts can be obtained from a balanced diet. However, threonine supplementation may be considered in certain cases, such as in athletes or individuals with specific medical conditions, to support protein synthesis, tissue repair, and overall health.

Overall, threonine is an essential amino acid that plays critical roles in protein synthesis, post-translational modifications, glycine and serine biosynthesis, mucin production, and collagen and elastin formation. Maintaining adequate intake of threonine through a balanced diet rich in protein sources is important for overall health and well-being.

Isoleucine is one of the nine essential amino acids, which means it cannot be synthesized by the body and must be obtained from the diet. *Here are some key points about isoleucine:*

- Amino Acid Structure: Isoleucine is an α-amino acid with a side chain that contains a methyl group and a branch, making it a branched-chain amino acid (BCAA). Its chemical structure includes an amino group (NH2), a carboxyl group (COOH), and a side chain containing a methyl group and a branched chain.

- Protein Synthesis: Isoleucine plays a crucial role in protein synthesis, where it is incorporated into proteins according to the genetic code. Along with leucine and valine, isoleucine is classified as a branched-chain amino acid (BCAA) and is involved in the synthesis of muscle proteins.

- Energy Metabolism: Isoleucine is involved in energy metabolism and can be oxidized for energy production in muscle tissue. During periods of prolonged exercise or fasting, isoleucine can be converted into acetyl-CoA and enter the citric acid cycle to generate ATP, the primary energy currency of cells.

- Muscle Protein Synthesis: Isoleucine, along with leucine and valine, plays a key role in stimulating muscle protein synthesis and promoting muscle growth and repair. BCAAs, including isoleucine, are preferentially taken up by muscle tissue and used as substrates for protein synthesis, particularly during and after exercise.

- Regulation of Blood Sugar: Isoleucine, along with leucine and valine, can help regulate blood sugar levels by stimulating the secretion of insulin, the hormone responsible for promoting glucose uptake by cells. BCAAs can enhance insulin sensitivity and glucose uptake in muscle tissue, which may help improve glycemic control and prevent insulin resistance.

- Brain Function: Isoleucine can cross the blood-brain barrier and is involved in neurotransmitter synthesis and brain function. It serves as a precursor for the synthesis of glutamate, an excitatory neurotransmitter, and GABA (gamma-aminobutyric acid), an inhibitory neurotransmitter, which play important roles in neuronal signaling and synaptic transmission.

- Dietary Sources: Isoleucine is found in a variety of protein-rich foods, particularly animal-based sources such as meat (such as beef, poultry, pork, and fish), eggs, dairy products (such as milk, cheese, and yogurt), and some plant-based sources such as soy products (such as tofu and tempeh), nuts, seeds, and legumes (such as beans and lentils).

- Supplementation: Isoleucine supplements are generally not necessary for most individuals, as adequate amounts can be obtained from a balanced diet. However, BCAA supplements containing isoleucine, leucine, and valine are sometimes used by athletes and individuals seeking to support muscle growth, recovery, and athletic performance.

Overall, isoleucine is an essential amino acid that plays critical roles in protein synthesis, energy metabolism, muscle function, blood sugar regulation, brain function, and overall health and well-being. Maintaining adequate intake of isoleucine through a balanced diet rich in protein sources is important for supporting various physiological processes in the body.

Leucine is one of the nine essential amino acids, which means it cannot be synthesized by the body and must be obtained from the diet. *Here are some key points about leucine*:

- Amino Acid Structure: Leucine is a α-amino acid with a side chain containing a methyl group and a branch, making it a branched-chain amino acid (BCAA). Its chemical structure includes an amino group (NH2), a carboxyl group (COOH), and a side chain containing a methyl group and a branched chain.

- Protein Synthesis: Leucine plays a crucial role in protein synthesis, where it is incorporated into proteins according to the genetic code. Along with isoleucine and valine, leucine is classified as a branched-chain amino acid (BCAA) and is involved in the synthesis of muscle proteins.
- Muscle Protein Synthesis: Leucine is particularly important for stimulating muscle protein synthesis and promoting muscle growth and repair. It activates the mammalian target of rapamycin (mTOR) signaling pathway, which is a key regulator of protein synthesis in muscle tissue. Higher levels of leucine in the blood can enhance TOR signaling and promote greater muscle protein synthesis.

- Regulation of Blood Sugar: Leucine can help regulate blood sugar levels by stimulating the secretion of insulin, the hormone responsible for promoting glucose uptake by cells. Leucine activates insulin signaling pathways in muscle tissue, which enhances glucose uptake and glycogen synthesis, leading to improved glycemic control.

- Energy Metabolism: Leucine is involved in energy metabolism and can be oxidized for energy production in muscle tissue. During periods of prolonged exercise or fasting, leucine can be converted into acetyl-CoA and enter the citric acid cycle to generate ATP, the primary energy currency of cells.

- Brain Function: Leucine can cross the blood-brain barrier and is involved in neurotransmitter synthesis and brain function. It serves as a precursor for the synthesis of glutamate, an excitatory neurotransmitter, and other neurotransmitters, which play important roles in neuronal signaling and synaptic transmission.

- Dietary Sources: Leucine is found in a variety of protein-rich foods, particularly animal-based sources such as meat (such as beef, poultry, pork, and fish), eggs, dairy products (such as milk, cheese, and yogurt), and some plant-based sources such as soy products (such as tofu and tempeh), nuts, seeds, and legumes (such as beans and lentils).

- Supplementation: Leucine supplements are sometimes used by athletes and individuals seeking to support muscle growth, recovery, and athletic performance. BCAA supplements containing leucine, isoleucine, and valine are also commonly used for these purposes, particularly before or after exercise to enhance muscle protein synthesis and reduce muscle damage.

Overall, leucine is an essential amino acid that plays critical roles in protein synthesis, muscle function, blood sugar regulation, energy metabolism, brain function, and overall health and well-being. Maintaining adequate intake of leucine through a balanced diet rich in protein sources is important for supporting various physiological processes in the body.

Valine is one of the nine essential amino acids, meaning it cannot be synthesized by the body and must be obtained from the diet. *Here are some key points about valine:*

- Amino Acid Structure: Valine is an α-amino acid with a side chain that contains a branched chain, making it a branched-chain amino acid (BCAA). Its chemical structure includes an amino group (NH2), a carboxyl group (COOH), and a side chain containing a methyl group and a branched chain.

- Protein Synthesis: Valine plays a vital role in protein synthesis, where it is incorporated into proteins according to the genetic code. Along with leucine and isoleucine, valine is classified as a branched-chain amino acid (BCAA), and it contributes to the synthesis of muscle proteins.

- Muscle Protein Synthesis: Valine, together with leucine and isoleucine, is involved in stimulating muscle protein synthesis and promoting muscle growth and repair. These BCAAs are preferentially taken up by muscle tissue and serve as substrates for protein synthesis, particularly during and after exercise.

- Energy Production: Valine can be oxidized for energy production in muscle tissue, particularly during periods of prolonged exercise or fasting. It can be converted into acetyl-CoA and enter the citric acid cycle to generate ATP, the primary energy currency of cells.

- Regulation of Blood Sugar: Valine, like leucine and isoleucine, can help regulate blood sugar levels by stimulating the secretion of insulin, the hormone responsible for promoting glucose uptake by cells. BCAAs can enhance insulin sensitivity and glucose uptake in muscle tissue, which may help improve glycemic control and prevent insulin resistance.

- Neurotransmitter Synthesis: Valine is involved in the synthesis of neurotransmitters such as GABA (gamma-amino butyric acid) and glutamate, which play important roles in neuronal signaling and brain function. Valine can cross the blood-brain barrier and contribute to neurotransmitter synthesis in the central nervous system.

- Dietary Sources: Valine is found in a variety of protein-rich foods, particularly animal-based sources such as meat (such as beef, poultry, pork, and fish), eggs, dairy products (such as milk, cheese, and yogurt), and some plant-based sources such as soy products (such as tofu and tempeh), nuts, seeds, and legumes (such as beans and lentils).

- Supplementation: Valine supplements are sometimes used by athletes and individuals seeking to support muscle growth, recovery, and athletic performance. BCAA supplements containing valine, leucine, and isoleucine are also commonly used for these purposes, particularly before or after exercise to enhance muscle protein synthesis and reduce muscle damage.

Overall, valine is an essential amino acid that plays critical roles in protein synthesis, muscle function, energy metabolism, blood sugar regulation, neurotransmitter synthesis, and overall health and well-being. Maintaining adequate intake of valine through a balanced diet rich in protein sources is important for supporting various physiological processes in the body.

Histidine is one of the twenty standard amino acids present in proteins. *Here are some key points about histidine:*

- Amino Acid Structure: Histidine is an α-amino acid, meaning that the amino group (NH2) is attached to the α-carbon atom of the molecule. It has a side chain containing an imidazole functional group, which is responsible for its unique chemical properties. The chemical structure of histidine includes an amino group (NH2), a carboxyl group (COOH), and a side chain containing an imidazole ring.

- Polarity: Histidine is classified as a polar amino acid due to the presence of the charged imidazole group in its side chain. This property makes it hydrophilic, meaning it has an affinity for water molecules.

- Essentiality: Histidine is considered semi-essential or conditionally essential because while the body can synthesize it, there are certain circumstances, such as during infancy or in individuals with certain metabolic disorders, where histidine must be obtained from the diet.

Biological Functions:

Histidine plays a crucial role in the structure and function of proteins. It can participate in hydrogen bonding interactions, contribute to protein stability, and be involved in enzyme catalysis and ligand binding.

- Histidine residues are often found in the active sites of enzymes, where they can act as proton donors or acceptors, facilitating enzyme-substrate interactions and catalytic reactions.

- Histidine serves as a precursor for the synthesis of important biological molecules, including histamine, an organic compound involved in immune responses, allergic reactions, and neurotransmission. Histidine is converted into histamine by the enzyme histidine decarboxylase.

- Histidine is also involved in metal ion coordination and binding. It can chelate metal ions such as zinc, copper, and iron, and participate in metalloproteinase structure and function.

- Dietary Sources: Histidine is found in a variety of protein-rich foods, particularly animal-based sources such as meat (such as beef, poultry, pork, and fish), eggs, dairy products (such as milk, cheese, and yogurt), and some plant-based sources such as soy products (such as tofu and tempeh), nuts, seeds, and legumes (such as beans and lentils).

- Health Implications: Histidine deficiency is rare in healthy individuals with a balanced diet, but it can occur in certain circumstances, such as during periods of rapid growth, illness, or inadequate protein intake. Histidine supplementation is generally not necessary for most people, but it may be considered in specific medical conditions or situations where histidine requirements are increased.

Overall, histidine is an important amino acid with diverse biological functions, including protein structure and function, enzyme catalysis, histamine synthesis, metal ion coordination, and overall health and well-being. Ensuring an adequate intake of histidine through a balanced diet rich in protein sources is essential for supporting various physiological processes in the body.

Arginine is a semi-essential or conditionally essential amino acid, meaning that while the body can typically produce it, there are certain circumstances where its production may be insufficient to meet the body's needs, necessitating dietary intake. *Here are some key points about arginine:*

- Amino Acid Structure: Arginine is an α-amino acid, containing an amino group (NH2) attached to the α-carbon atom, a carboxyl group (COOH), and a side chain containing a guanidinium group. Its chemical structure includes a basic amino group and a positively charged guanidinium group, which confer unique properties to arginine.

Biological Functions:

- Arginine serves as a precursor for the synthesis of nitric oxide (NO), a signaling molecule involved in various physiological processes such as vasodilation, neurotransmission, immune function, and inflammation. Nitric oxide helps regulate blood flow, blood pressure, and vascular tone by relaxing smooth muscle cells in blood vessels.

- Arginine is involved in protein synthesis and cellular growth, as it is incorporated into proteins according to the genetic code. It plays a role in the synthesis of various proteins, including enzymes, structural proteins, and signaling molecules.

- Arginine is important for the urea cycle, a metabolic pathway in the liver that converts toxic ammonia into urea for excretion. Arginine acts as a substrate for the enzyme arginase, which catalyzes the final step of the urea cycle, producing urea and ornithine.

- Arginine plays a role in immune function and wound healing, as it is involved in the synthesis of polyamines, which are essential for cell proliferation and tissue repair. Arginine supplementation may help support immune function and enhance wound healing in certain situations.

- Dietary Sources: Arginine is found in a variety of protein-rich foods, particularly animal-based sources such as meat (such as beef, poultry, pork, and fish), dairy products (such as milk, cheese, and yogurt), eggs, and some plant-based sources such as nuts, seeds, soy products (such as tofu and tempeh), and legumes (such as beans and lentils).

Health Implications:

- Arginine deficiency is rare in healthy individuals with a balanced diet, as the body can typically synthesize arginine from other amino acids, particularly glutamine, glutamate, and proline. However, arginine synthesis may be impaired in certain conditions such as sepsis, trauma, burns, or during periods of rapid growth.

- Arginine supplementation has been studied for various health conditions, including cardiovascular disease, erectile dysfunction, athletic performance, and immune function. While some studies have shown potential benefits of arginine supplementation in certain contexts, more research is needed to fully understand its effects and determine optimal dosages.

Overall, arginine is an important amino acid with diverse biological functions, including nitric oxide synthesis, protein synthesis, urea cycle metabolism, immune function, and wound healing. Ensuring an adequate intake of arginine through a balanced diet rich in protein sources is important for supporting various physiological processes in the body.

COENZYME

Nicotinamide, also known as niacinamide or vitamin B3, is a water-soluble vitamin and essential nutrient that plays crucial roles in various physiological processes in the body. *Here are some key points about nicotinamide:*

- Vitamin B3: Nicotinamide is one of the two primary forms of vitamin B3, the other being nicotinic acid. It is an essential nutrient, meaning that it must be obtained from the diet as the body cannot synthesize it in sufficient amounts. Nicotinamide is converted into its active coenzyme forms, nicotinamide adenine dinucleotide (NAD+) and nicotinamide adenine dinucleotide phosphate (NADP+), which serve as cofactors for numerous enzymatic reactions in the body.

Biological Functions:

- Energy metabolism: Nicotinamide participates in cellular energy production through its involvement in the metabolism of carbohydrates, fats, and proteins. It serves as a coenzyme for several key enzymes involved in glycolysis, the tricarboxylic acid (TCA) cycle, and oxidative phosphorylation, which are processes that generate ATP, the body's primary energy currency.

- Redox reactions: Nicotinamide functions as a cofactor for enzymes involved in redox reactions, which are chemical reactions that involve the transfer of electrons. NAD+ and NADP+ serve as electron carriers, accepting and donating electrons during metabolic processes such as cellular respiration, fatty acid oxidation, and antioxidant defense.

- DNA repair and maintenance: Nicotinamide plays a role in DNA repair mechanisms and helps maintain genomic stability. It is involved in the activity of enzymes called poly(ADP-ribose) polymerases (PARPs), which are important for repairing DNA damage caused by various factors such as oxidative stress, radiation, and genotoxic agents.

- Gene expression regulation: Nicotinamide influences gene expression patterns by acting as a substrate for enzymes known as sirtuins, which are a class of NAD+-dependent protein deacetylases. Sirtuins play roles in various cellular processes, including metabolism, aging, and stress response, by modifying the activity of histones and other proteins through deacetylation.

- Skin health: Nicotinamide has been shown to have beneficial effects on skin health and is commonly used in skincare products for its anti-inflammatory, antioxidant, and moisturizing properties. It can help improve the appearance of aging skin, reduce the risk of skin cancer, and alleviate symptoms of certain skin conditions such as acne, rosacea, and eczema.

- Dietary Sources: Nicotinamide is found in a variety of foods, particularly animal-based sources such as meat (such as poultry, beef, and fish), eggs, and dairy products (such as milk and cheese). It is also present in plant-based sources such as nuts, seeds, legumes, whole grains, and fortified cereals. Additionally, nicotinamide can be synthesized in the body from the amino acid tryptophan, although this pathway may not always provide sufficient amounts to meet daily requirements.

Health Implications:

- Nicotinamide deficiency can lead to a condition known as pellagra, characterized by symptoms such as skin rash, diarrhea, dementia, and eventually death if left untreated. Pellagra is rare in developed countries due to the widespread availability of niacin-rich foods and niacin fortification of staple foods such as flour and cornmeal.

- Nicotinamide supplementation may be recommended for certain medical conditions or situations where there is an increased demand for vitamin B3, such as in individuals with niacin deficiency, metabolic disorders, or certain skin conditions. However, excessive nicotinamide intake can lead to adverse effects such as flushing, liver toxicity, and insulin resistance.

Overall, nicotinamide is an essential nutrient that plays critical roles in energy metabolism, redox reactions, DNA repair, gene expression regulation, and skin health. Ensuring an adequate intake of nicotinamide through a balanced diet and, if necessary, supplementation is important for supporting overall health and well-being.

Biotin, also known as vitamin B7 or vitamin H is a water-soluble vitamin that plays a key role in various metabolic processes in the body. *Here are some key points about biotin:*

- Coenzyme: Biotin serves as a coenzyme for several carboxylase enzymes involved in important metabolic pathways. These enzymes add a carboxyl group to substrates, which is essential for the synthesis of fatty acids, amino acids, and glucose, as well as for the metabolism of certain amino acids and fatty acids.
- Carboxylase Enzymes: Biotin is a cofactor for the following carboxylase enzymes:

- Acetyl-CoA carboxylase: This enzyme is involved in the synthesis of fatty acids from acetyl-CoA, a process important for the production of lipids needed for cellular membranes, energy storage, and signaling molecules.

- Propionyl-CoA carboxylase: This enzyme is involved in the metabolism of certain amino acids and fatty acids, particularly branched-chain amino acids and odd-chain fatty acids. It helps convert propionyl-CoA into methylmalonyl-CoA, which can then enter the TCA cycle for energy production or be converted into succinyl-CoA for heme synthesis.

- Pyruvate carboxylase: This enzyme is involved in gluconeogenesis, the synthesis of glucose from non-carbohydrate precursors such as amino acids and lactate. It helps convert pyruvate into oxaloacetate, a key intermediate in gluconeogenesis.

- Metabolic Functions: Biotin plays a crucial role in various metabolic processes, including:

- Fatty acid synthesis: Biotin is essential for the synthesis of fatty acids, which are important for energy storage, membrane structure, and cellular signaling.

- Gluconeogenesis: Biotin is required for the conversion of certain substrates into glucose, particularly during periods of fasting or low carbohydrate intake when glucose availability is limited.

- Amino acid metabolism: Biotin is involved in the breakdown and utilization of amino acids, particularly those with sulfur-containing side chains such as methionine and cysteine.

- Hair, Skin, and Nail Health: Biotin is often promoted for its potential benefits for hair, skin, and nail health. While scientific evidence supporting these claims is limited, biotin deficiency can lead to symptoms such as hair loss, dermatitis, and brittle nails. Biotin supplementation may be recommended for individuals with biotin deficiency or certain medical conditions affecting hair, skin, and nails.

- Dietary Sources: Biotin is found in a variety of foods, particularly protein-rich sources such as egg yolks, liver, nuts, seeds, legumes, and certain vegetables (such as sweet potatoes and leafy greens). Biotin is also produced by bacteria in the gut, although the extent to which this contributes to overall biotin status is unclear.

- Deficiency: Biotin deficiency is rare, as biotin is widely available in foods and is also synthesized by gut bacteria. However, certain factors such as prolonged antibiotic use, excessive consumption of raw egg whites (which contain avidin, a protein that binds biotin and prevents its absorption), and certain genetic disorders affecting biotin metabolism can increase the risk of deficiency. Symptoms of biotin deficiency may include hair loss, skin rash, neurological abnormalities, and metabolic disturbances.

- Supplementation: Biotin supplementation is commonly used for hair, skin, and nail health, as well as for certain medical conditions such as biotinidase deficiency and metabolic disorders affecting biotin metabolism. Biotin supplements are generally considered safe when taken at recommended doses, although high doses may cause adverse effects such as gastrointestinal symptoms and interference with laboratory tests.

Overall, biotin is an essential vitamin that plays critical roles in various metabolic processes in the body, particularly fatty acid synthesis, gluconeogenesis, and amino acid metabolism. Ensuring an adequate intake of biotin through a balanced diet and, if necessary, supplementation is important for supporting overall health and well-being.

Pantothenic acid, also known as vitamin B5, is a water-soluble vitamin that plays a crucial role in various metabolic processes in the body. *Here are some key points about pantothenic acid:*

- Coenzyme A (CoA) Synthesis: Pantothenic acid is a precursor for coenzyme A (CoA), a coenzyme that plays a central role in numerous metabolic pathways. CoA is essential for the synthesis and oxidation of fatty acids, the synthesis of cholesterol, the metabolism of carbohydrates and amino acids, and the production of acetylcholine, a neurotransmitter.

- Acetyl-CoA Formation: Pantothenic acid is a component of CoA, which functions as an acyl group carrier in many metabolic reactions. Acetyl-CoA, the activated form of acetic acid, is generated from the breakdown of carbohydrates, fats, and proteins. It serves as a substrate for the tricarboxylic acid (TCA) cycle, where it undergoes oxidation to produce energy in the form of ATP.

- Fatty Acid Synthesis: Pantothenic acid is essential for the synthesis of fatty acids, which are building blocks for various lipids such as phospholipids, triglycerides, and cholesterol esters. CoA serves as an acyl carrier in the synthesis of fatty acids, facilitating the stepwise addition of acetyl and malonyl groups during fatty acid elongation.

- Cholesterol Synthesis: Pantothenic acid is involved in the synthesis of cholesterol, a vital component of cell membranes and a precursor for steroid hormones, bile acids, and vitamin D. CoA is required for the conversion of acetyl-CoA into mevalonate, the initial step in the cholesterol biosynthesis pathway.

- Amino Acid Metabolism: Pantothenic acid is necessary for the metabolism of amino acids, particularly the conversion of branched-chain amino acids (leucine, isoleucine, and valine) into their respective acyl-CoA derivatives.

These acyl-CoA compounds can then enter the TCA cycle for energy production or be used for the synthesis of other biomolecules.

- Hemoglobin Synthesis: Pantothenic acid is involved in the synthesis of heme, the iron-containing component of hemoglobin, the oxygen-carrying protein in red blood cells. CoA is required for the conversion of succinyl-CoA into δ-aminolevulinic acid (ALA), an intermediate in the heme biosynthesis pathway.

- Dietary Sources: Pantothenic acid is found in a variety of foods, particularly animal-based sources such as meat (such as beef, poultry, pork, and fish), eggs, dairy products (such as milk, cheese, and yogurt), and organ meats (such as liver and kidney). It is also present in plant-based sources such as whole grains, legumes, nuts, seeds, and certain vegetables (such as avocados and mushrooms).

- Deficiency: Pantothenic acid deficiency is rare, as it is widely available in many foods. However, severe deficiencies can occur in individuals with malabsorption disorders, chronic alcoholism, or certain metabolic disorders affecting pantothenic acid metabolism. Symptoms of deficiency may include fatigue, irritability, numbness and tingling in the extremities, gastrointestinal disturbances, and impaired wound healing.

- Supplementation: Pantothenic acid supplements are available and are sometimes used for the treatment of certain medical conditions or as a component of multivitamin and B-complex formulations. However, supplementation is generally not necessary for individuals with a balanced diet, as pantothenic acid requirements can typically be met through food sources.

Overall, pantothenic acid is an essential vitamin that plays critical roles in energy metabolism, fatty acid synthesis, cholesterol synthesis, amino acid metabolism, and hemoglobin synthesis. Ensuring an adequate intake of pantothenic acid through a balanced diet is important for supporting overall health and well-being.

Folic acid, also known as folate or vitamin B9, is a water-soluble vitamin that plays a crucial role in various physiological processes in the body. *Here are some key points about folic acid:*

- DNA Synthesis and Repair: Folic acid is essential for the synthesis and repair of DNA, the genetic material found in every cell of the body. It is involved in the synthesis of nucleotides, the building blocks of DNA, which are necessary for cell division, growth, and tissue repair. Folic acid participates in the conversion of deoxyuridine monophosphate (dUMP) into deoxythymidine monophosphate (dTMP), a precursor for thymidine, one of the four nucleotides in DNA.

- Cell Division and Growth: Folic acid is important for cell division and growth, particularly during periods of rapid cell proliferation such as embryonic development, infancy, and pregnancy. Adequate folic acid intake is essential for normal fetal development, as it is required for the formation of the neural tube, which develops into the brain and spinal cord of the embryo.

- Red Blood Cell Formation: Folic acid is necessary for the maturation of red blood cells (erythropoiesis) and the synthesis of hemoglobin, the oxygen-carrying protein in red blood cells. Folic acid deficiency can lead to megaloblastic anemia; a type of anemia characterized by large, immature red blood cells (megaloblasts) and reduced hemoglobin levels.

- Amino Acid Metabolism: Folic acid is involved in the metabolism of certain amino acids, particularly methionine and homocysteine. It serves as a cofactor for enzymes involved in the remethylation of homocysteine to methionine, a process that requires vitamin B12 as well. Elevated levels of homocysteine due to folic acid deficiency have been associated with an increased risk of cardiovascular disease.

- Neurological Function: Folic acid is important for maintaining optimal neurological function, as it is involved in the synthesis of neurotransmitters such as serotonin, dopamine, and norepinephrine. Adequate folic acid intake may help support cognitive function, mood regulation, and mental health.

- Dietary Sources: Folic acid is found in a variety of foods, particularly green leafy vegetables (such as spinach, kale, and broccoli), legumes (such as beans, lentils, and peas), fruits (such as oranges and avocados), nuts, seeds, whole grains, fortified cereals, and animal-based sources such as liver and eggs. Fortified foods, such as breakfast cereals and grain products, are also significant sources of folic acid.

- Supplementation: Folic acid supplementation is recommended for certain populations, particularly women of childbearing age, pregnant women, and individuals with conditions that increase the risk of folic acid deficiency (such as malabsorption disorders, alcoholism, or certain medications). Folic acid supplements are commonly used to prevent neural tube defects (such as spina bifida) and other birth defects during pregnancy.

- Health Implications: Folic acid deficiency can lead to various health problems, including megaloblastic anemia, neural tube defects, cardiovascular disease, and neurological disorders. Adequate folic acid intake is important for overall health and well-being, particularly during pregnancy and periods of rapid growth and development.

Overall, folic acid is an essential vitamin that plays critical roles in DNA synthesis and repair, cell division and growth, red blood cell formation, amino acid metabolism, neurological function, and overall health. Ensuring an adequate intake of folic acid through a balanced diet and, if necessary, supplementation is important for supporting various physiological processes in the body.

Coenzyme Q10 (CoQ10), also known as ubiquinone, is a naturally occurring compound found in the mitochondria of cells throughout the body. *Here are some key points about Coenzyme Q10:*

- Biological Role: CoQ10 plays a crucial role in cellular energy production. It is a component of the electron transport chain, a series of protein complexes located in the inner mitochondrial membrane that generate adenosine triphosphate (ATP), the primary energy currency of cells. CoQ10 acts as an electron carrier, shuttling electrons between complex I and complex III of the electron transport chain, which ultimately leads to the production of ATP.

- Antioxidant Properties: CoQ10 also has antioxidant properties, meaning it can neutralize harmful free radicals and reduce oxidative stress in cells. Free radicals are highly reactive molecules that can damage cell membranes, proteins, and DNA, contributing to various age-related diseases and conditions such as cardiovascular disease, neurodegenerative disorders, and cancer. CoQ10 helps protect cells from oxidative damage by scavenging free radicals and regenerating other antioxidants such as vitamin E.

- Endogenous Synthesis: While CoQ10 can be obtained from dietary sources, the majority of CoQ10 in the body is synthesized endogenously, primarily in the liver. The biosynthesis of CoQ10 involves multiple steps and requires various enzymes and cofactors. Coenzyme Q10 synthesis can be influenced by factors such as age, genetics, dietary intake of precursor nutrients, and certain medical conditions.

- Dietary Sources: CoQ10 is found in small amounts in certain foods, particularly organ meats (such as liver, heart, and kidney), beef, pork, poultry, fatty fish (such as salmon, mackerel, and sardines), and vegetable oils (such as soybean and canola oil). While dietary sources can contribute to CoQ10 intake, most of the CoQ10 in the body is synthesized endogenously.

- Supplementation: CoQ10 supplements are available and are commonly used for various health purposes, including:

- Supporting cardiovascular health: CoQ10 supplementation may help improve heart function, reduce blood pressure, and enhance exercise performance in individuals with heart failure, hypertension, or other cardiovascular conditions.

- Supporting mitochondrial function: CoQ10 supplementation may benefit individuals with mitochondrial disorders, which are genetic or acquired conditions characterized by impaired energy production and oxidative stress.

- Anti-aging and antioxidant effects: CoQ10 supplementation may help reduce oxidative damage, enhance cellular energy production, and support overall health and longevity.

- Health Implications: CoQ10 deficiency is rare, as the body can synthesize CoQ10 and obtain it from dietary sources. However, certain factors such as aging, genetic mutations, certain medications (such as statins), and medical conditions (such as mitochondrial disorders or heart failure) can lead to decreased CoQ10 levels or impaired CoQ10 function. CoQ10 supplementation may be beneficial in these cases to restore CoQ10 levels and support cellular energy production and antioxidant defense.

Overall, Coenzyme Q10 is a vital compound involved in cellular energy production and antioxidant defense. While the body can synthesize CoQ10 and obtain it from dietary sources, supplementation may be beneficial for certain individuals to support cardiovascular health, mitochondrial function, and overall well-being. As with any supplement, it's important to consult with a healthcare professional before starting CoQ10 supplementation, especially if you have underlying medical conditions or are taking medications.

Glutathione is a powerful antioxidant and tripeptide molecule composed of three amino acids: glutamine, cysteine, and glycine. It is found in virtually every cell in the body and plays several essential roles in maintaining overall health. *Here are some key points about glutathione:*

- Antioxidant Defense: Glutathione is one of the body's primary antioxidants, meaning it helps neutralize harmful free radicals and reactive oxygen species (ROS) that can damage cells and contribute to oxidative stress. It accomplishes this by donating electrons to neutralize free radicals, thereby protecting cells from oxidative damage and maintaining their integrity.

- Detoxification: Glutathione is a key player in the body's detoxification processes, particularly in the liver. It acts as a cofactor for various enzymes involved in detoxifying and eliminating harmful substances, including environmental toxins, heavy metals, drugs, and metabolic byproducts.

Glutathione conjugates with toxins to make them water-soluble, allowing for their excretion via urine or bile.

- Immune Function: Glutathione plays a critical role in supporting the immune system's function. It helps regulate the activity of immune cells, such as lymphocytes and macrophages, and promotes the production of cytokines, which are signaling molecules involved in immune responses. Glutathione deficiency has been associated with impaired immune function and increased susceptibility to infections and inflammatory conditions.

- Antioxidant Recycling: Glutathione acts as a recycling agent for other antioxidants, such as vitamin C and vitamin E. After these antioxidants neutralize free radicals, they become oxidized themselves. Glutathione helps regenerate them back to their active forms, allowing them to continue their antioxidant activities and prolonging their effectiveness in protecting cells from oxidative damage.

- Cellular Defense and Repair: Glutathione plays a crucial role in maintaining cellular health and integrity. It helps protect cellular components such as proteins, lipids, and DNA from oxidative damage, thereby preserving cellular function and preventing premature aging. Glutathione also supports DNA repair mechanisms, helping to maintain genomic stability and integrity.

- Dietary Sources: While glutathione is present in many foods, it is not effectively absorbed intact by the body when consumed orally. Instead, the body relies on the synthesis of glutathione from its precursor amino acids, particularly cysteine. Foods rich in cysteine, such as eggs, poultry, dairy products, nuts, seeds, and legumes, can support glutathione synthesis.

- Supplementation: Glutathione supplements are available and are used for various purposes, including supporting antioxidant defense, detoxification, immune function, and overall health. However, the effectiveness of oral glutathione supplementation is debated, as it is not well absorbed by the body and may be broken down in the digestive tract. Some studies suggest that certain forms of glutathione supplements, such as liposomal or acetylated glutathione, may have better bioavailability.

Overall, glutathione is a critical molecule with diverse functions in the body, including antioxidant defense, detoxification, immune support, and cellular health. Maintaining optimal glutathione levels through dietary sources of its precursor amino acids and supporting its synthesis may help promote overall health and protect against oxidative stress-related diseases and conditions.

FATTY ACID

Linoleic acid is an essential omega-6 fatty acid, meaning that it cannot be synthesized by the human body and must be obtained from the diet. It is a polyunsaturated fatty acid (PUFA) with 18 carbon atoms and two double bonds, and it is a precursor to other important omega-6 fatty acids, such as arachidonic acid.

Here are some key points about linoleic acid:

- Structural Role: Linoleic acid is a major component of cell membranes and is essential for maintaining their fluidity and integrity. It helps form the lipid bilayer that surrounds cells, providing structural support and regulating the movement of molecules in and out of the cell.

- Precursor to Bioactive Molecules: Linoleic acid serves as a precursor for the synthesis of other biologically active compounds, including arachidonic acid, which is further metabolized into various eicosanoids such as prostaglandins, thromboxane, and leukotriene. These eicosanoids play crucial roles in inflammation, immune response, blood clotting, and vascular tone regulation.

- Skin Health: Linoleic acid is important for maintaining healthy skin. It helps strengthen the skin barrier, retain moisture, and prevent transepidermal water loss, which can help reduce dryness, inflammation, and signs of aging such as wrinkles and fine lines. Linoleic acid deficiency may contribute to skin disorders such as atopic dermatitis and acne.

- Cardiovascular Health: Linoleic acid, along with other polyunsaturated fatty acids, has been associated with cardiovascular benefits. It can help lower levels of low-density lipoprotein (LDL) cholesterol, reduce inflammation, and improve endothelial function, which may lower the risk of heart disease and stroke.

- Dietary Sources: Linoleic acid is found in various plant-based oils, seeds, nuts, and their derived products. Some of the richest dietary sources include sunflower oil, safflower oil, soybean oil, corn oil, cottonseed oil, sesame oil, and pumpkin seeds. Consuming a balanced diet that includes these sources can help ensure an adequate intake of linoleic acid.

- Recommended Intake: The recommended daily intake of linoleic acid varies depending on age, sex, and specific health conditions. In general, adults should aim to consume about 5-10% of their total daily calories from linoleic acid, according to dietary guidelines. However, excessive consumption of omega-6 fatty acids relative to omega-3 fatty acids may have adverse health effects, so it's important to maintain a balanced ratio between the two.

Overall, linoleic acid is an essential nutrient with important roles in cell structure, skin health, cardiovascular function, and inflammation regulation. Including sources of linoleic acid in the diet can contribute to overall health and well-being, but moderation and balance are key to optimizing its benefits.

Arachidonic acid (AA) is a polyunsaturated omega-6 fatty acid with 20 carbon atoms and four double bonds. It is found in cell membranes throughout the body and is particularly abundant in the brain, muscles, liver, and adipose tissue. Arachidonic acid is synthesized from linoleic acid, an essential omega-6 fatty acid, through the action of enzymes called desaturases and elongates.

Here are some key points about arachidonic acid:

- Biological Role: Arachidonic acid serves as a precursor for the synthesis of various biologically active molecules called eicosanoids. Eicosanoids are signaling molecules that play important roles in inflammation, immune response, blood clotting, and vascular tone regulation. Some examples of eicosanoids derived from arachidonic acid include prostaglandins, thromboxane, and leukotriene.

- Inflammatory Response: Arachidonic acid metabolism is closely linked to the body's inflammatory response. When cells are stimulated by injury, infection, or other stimuli, arachidonic acid is released from cell membranes and converted into prostaglandins and leukotriene by specific enzymes called cyclooxygenases (COX) and lipoxygenases (LOX), respectively. These eicosanoids promote inflammation by inducing vasodilation, increasing vascular permeability, and recruiting immune cells to the site of injury or infection.

- Regulation of Physiological Processes: Eicosanoids derived from arachidonic acid play diverse roles in regulating physiological processes throughout the body. For example:

Prostaglandins help regulate blood pressure, kidney function, gastrointestinal motility, and female reproductive function (such as inducing uterine contractions during childbirth).

Thromboxane promotes platelet aggregation and blood clot formation, contributing to hemostasis and wound healing.

Leukotriene are involved in allergic and inflammatory responses, particularly in the respiratory system, where they can cause bronchoconstriction and mucus production.

- Dietary Sources: While arachidonic acid can be synthesized endogenously from linoleic acid, it is also found in certain animal-based foods. Some dietary sources of arachidonic acid include meat (particularly red meat and organ meats), poultry, eggs, and fish. Consumption of these foods can contribute to arachidonic acid intake in the diet.

- Health Implications: The role of arachidonic acid in inflammation and immune response has led to interest in its potential role in various health conditions, including cardiovascular disease, inflammatory disorders, and neurodegenerative diseases. While some studies suggest that excessive intake of arachidonic acid or imbalance in the ratio of omega-6 to omega-3 fatty acids may contribute to inflammation and chronic disease risk, more research is needed to fully understand its effects and implications for health.

Overall, arachidonic acid is an important fatty acid with diverse biological functions in the body. While it plays critical roles in inflammation, immune response, and physiological regulation, maintaining a balanced intake of omega-6 and omega-3 fatty acids is essential for optimal health and well-being.

ENDOCRINE SYSTEM

Thyroid hormones, primarily thyroxine (T4) and triiodothyronine (T3), are produced and secreted by the thyroid gland and play essential roles in regulating metabolism, growth, and development.

Here are some common indices and tests used to evaluate thyroid function:

- Thyroid Stimulating Hormone (TSH): TSH is produced by the pituitary gland and stimulates the thyroid gland to produce and release T4 and T3. TSH levels are often measured as part of thyroid function tests to assess thyroid gland activity. Elevated TSH levels may indicate hypothyroidism (underactive thyroid), while low TSH levels may indicate hyperthyroidism (overactive thyroid).

- Free Thyroxine (FT4) and Free Triiodothyronine (FT3): FT4 and FT3 are the active forms of thyroid hormones that are not bound to proteins in the blood and are available for use by the body's cells. Measurement of FT4 and FT3 levels provides information about the actual amount of thyroid hormone circulating in the bloodstream and can help diagnose thyroid disorders.

- Total T4 and Total T3: These tests measure the total amount of T4 and T3 in the blood, including both protein-bound and free forms. While total T4 and T3 levels can provide useful information about thyroid function, they may be influenced by changes in protein levels and binding capacity in the blood.

- Thyroid Antibody Tests: These tests measure the levels of antibodies produced by the immune system that target components of the thyroid gland, such as thyroid peroxidase antibodies (TPOAb) and thyroglobulin antibodies (TgAb). Elevated antibody levels may indicate autoimmune thyroid conditions such as Hashimoto's thyroiditis or Graves' disease.

- Thyroid Ultrasound: Ultrasound imaging of the thyroid gland can provide information about its size, structure, and the presence of nodules or abnormalities. This imaging modality is often used to evaluate thyroid nodules and assess for signs of thyroiditis or other thyroid disorders.

- Thyroid Uptake and Scan: This nuclear medicine test involves the administration of a radioactive tracer, followed by imaging to assess the thyroid gland's ability to take up and retain iodine. Thyroid uptake and scan can help diagnose conditions such as hyperthyroidism, thyroid nodules, or thyroid cancer.

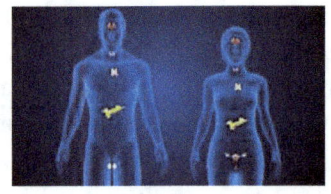

It's important to note that interpretation of thyroid function tests should be done in consultation with a healthcare professional, as multiple factors can influence test results, and individual patient characteristics must be considered for accurate diagnosis and management of thyroid disorders.

The parathyroid glands are small endocrine glands located near the thyroid gland in the neck. Their primary function is to regulate calcium and phosphate levels in the blood through the secretion of parathyroid hormone (PTH). PTH plays a crucial role in calcium homeostasis by increasing calcium levels in the blood through several mechanisms, including increasing calcium absorption from the intestines, releasing calcium from bones, and promoting calcium reabsorption in the kidneys while enhancing phosphate

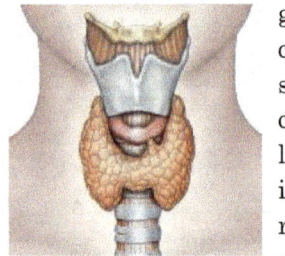

excretion.

Here are some common tests and parameters used to assess parathyroid gland function and PTH secretion:

- Serum Parathyroid Hormone (PTH) Levels: Measurement of PTH levels in the blood can provide information about parathyroid gland activity. Elevated PTH levels may indicate primary hyperparathyroidism, a condition characterized by excessive PTH secretion due to benign tumors or hyperplasia of the parathyroid glands. Conversely, low PTH levels may indicate hyperparathyroidism, which can occur due to damage or dysfunction of the parathyroid glands.

- Serum Calcium Levels: PTH secretion is regulated by changes in serum calcium levels. When calcium levels in the blood are low, the parathyroid glands secrete more PTH to stimulate calcium release from bones and increase calcium absorption from the intestines and kidneys. Conversely, when calcium levels are high, PTH secretion is suppressed. Therefore, measuring serum calcium levels alongside PTH levels can help evaluate parathyroid gland function and calcium homeostasis.

- Serum Phosphate Levels: PTH also plays a role in phosphate homeostasis, although its effects on phosphate levels are less pronounced compared to calcium. PTH decreases phosphate levels in the blood by promoting phosphate excretion in the kidneys. Therefore, measurement of serum phosphate levels can provide additional information about parathyroid gland function and calcium-phosphate balance.

- Bone Mineral Density (BMD) Testing: In cases of primary hyperparathyroidism, excessive PTH secretion can lead to increased bone resorption and loss of bone mineral density, potentially resulting in osteoporosis or osteopenia. Bone mineral density testing using dual-energy X-ray absorptiometry (DXA) can help assess bone health and detect changes in bone density associated with hyperparathyroidism.

- Imaging Studies: Imaging modalities such as ultrasound, computed tomography (CT), or nuclear medicine scans may be used to visualize the parathyroid glands and detect abnormalities such as adenomas or hyperplasia, which can cause hyperparathyroidism.

Overall, assessing parathyroid gland function and PTH secretion involves a combination of clinical evaluation, laboratory tests, and imaging studies to diagnose and manage conditions affecting calcium and phosphate metabolism, such as hyperparathyroidism and hyperparathyroidism. Treatment options may include medication, surgery, or other interventions aimed at restoring normal parathyroid gland function and calcium homeostasis.

The adrenal glands are vital endocrine glands located above the kidneys, responsible for producing several hormones essential for regulating various physiological processes in the body. These hormones include cortisol, aldosterone, adrenaline (epinephrine), and noradrenaline (norepinephrine).

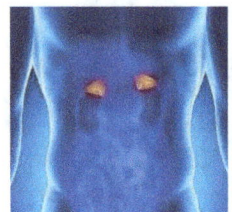

Here are some common assessments related to adrenal gland function:

- Hormone Testing: Hormone levels produced by the adrenal glands can be evaluated through blood or urine tests. This includes measuring cortisol levels to assess adrenal function and screen for conditions such as Cushing's syndrome (excess cortisol) or Addison's disease (adrenal insufficiency). Aldosterone levels may also be measured to evaluate adrenal function in regulating electrolyte balance and blood pressure.

- ACTH Stimulation Test: This test evaluates the adrenal glands' ability to respond to adrenocorticotropic hormone (ACTH) stimulation by measuring cortisol levels before and after administration of synthetic ACTH. It helps diagnose conditions such as adrenal insufficiency and evaluates the adrenal glands' responsiveness to ACTH stimulation.

- Imaging Studies: Imaging modalities such as computed tomography (CT) scan or magnetic resonance imaging (MRI) may be used to visualize the adrenal glands and detect abnormalities such as tumors or nodules. This can help diagnose conditions such as adrenal tumors, adrenal hyperplasia, or adrenal gland enlargement.

- Adrenal Antibody Testing: In cases of autoimmune conditions affecting the adrenal glands, such as autoimmune adrenalitis (Addison's disease), specific antibodies targeting adrenal tissue may be detected through blood tests. This can aid in the diagnosis and management of autoimmune adrenal disorders.

- Dexamethasone Suppression Test: This test evaluates the adrenal glands' response to synthetic glucocorticoid medication (dexamethasone) by measuring cortisol levels before and after administration. It helps diagnose conditions such as Cushing's syndrome and assesses the feedback regulation of cortisol production by the hypothalamic-pituitary-adrenal (HPA) axis.

- 24-Hour Urinary Free Cortisol Test: This test measures cortisol levels in a 24-hour urine collection sample and is used to assess cortisol production over an extended period. It is often performed to evaluate conditions such as Cushing's syndrome, where excess cortisol production is suspected.

Evaluation of adrenal gland function may vary depending on the clinical presentation and suspected underlying conditions. Healthcare providers may use a combination of history taking, physical examination, laboratory tests, and imaging studies to assess adrenal gland health and function accurately. If you have concerns about your adrenal gland function, it's essential to consult with a healthcare professional for proper evaluation and management.

The pituitary gland, often referred to as the "master gland," is a crucial component of the endocrine system and plays a vital role in regulating various physiological processes in the body by secreting hormones. These hormones act on target organs and glands to control growth, metabolism, reproduction, stress response, and other functions.

Here are some common assessments related to pituitary gland function:

- Hormone Testing: Hormone levels secreted by the pituitary gland can be evaluated through blood tests. The pituitary gland secretes several hormones, including:

- Growth Hormone (GH): Regulates growth and metabolism.

- Adrenocorticotropic Hormone (ACTH): Stimulates the adrenal glands to produce cortisol and other adrenal hormones.

- Thyroid-Stimulating Hormone (TSH): Stimulates the thyroid gland to produce thyroid hormones.
- Luteinizing Hormone (LH) and Follicle-Stimulating Hormone (FSH): Regulate reproductive function in both males and females.

- Prolactin: Stimulates milk production in lactating women.

- Antidiuretic Hormone (ADH), also known as Vasopressin: Regulates water balance and blood pressure.

- Oxytocin: Involved in labor and breastfeeding.

- Stimulation Tests: Stimulation tests may be performed to assess the pituitary gland's ability to respond to certain stimuli. For example, a growth hormone stimulation test involves administering agents that stimulate GH secretion, followed by blood tests to measure GH levels. This test can help diagnose growth hormone deficiency or excess.

- Suppression Tests: Suppression tests may be used to assess the pituitary glands feedback mechanisms. For instance, a dexamethasone suppression test evaluates the pituitary-adrenal axis by administering a synthetic glucocorticoid (dexamethasone) to suppress cortisol production. This test can help diagnose conditions such as Cushing's syndrome.

- Imaging Studies: Imaging modalities such as magnetic resonance imaging (MRI) or computed tomography (CT) scans may be used to visualize the pituitary gland and detect abnormalities such as tumors, cysts, or structural changes. These imaging studies can aid in the diagnosis of conditions affecting pituitary function, such as pituitary adenomas.

- Visual Field Testing: In cases of pituitary tumors that may compress surrounding structures, such as the optic nerves, visual field testing may be performed to assess for potential visual field defects or abnormalities.

Evaluation of pituitary gland function may vary depending on the clinical presentation and suspected underlying conditions. Healthcare providers may use a combination of history taking, physical examination, laboratory tests, and imaging studies to assess pituitary gland health and function accurately. If you have concerns about your pituitary gland function, it's essential to consult with a healthcare professional for proper evaluation and management.

The pineal gland, a small endocrine gland located in the brain, secretes the hormone melatonin, which plays a crucial role in regulating the sleep-wake cycle (circadian rhythm) and other physiological functions. Melatonin secretion by the pineal gland is influenced by environmental factors such as light and darkness.

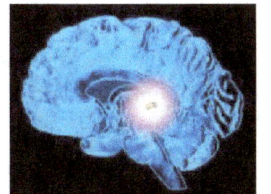

Healthcare professionals may assess pineal function and melatonin levels through various methods:

- Melatonin Levels: Melatonin levels in the blood or saliva can be measured to assess pineal gland function. Melatonin secretion typically follows a circadian rhythm, with higher levels at night (in response to darkness) and lower levels during the day. Measurement of melatonin levels may be useful in diagnosing sleep disorders, circadian rhythm disorders, or evaluating the effects of light exposure on melatonin secretion.

- 24-Hour Urinary Melatonin Excretion: Some studies measure the amount of melatonin excreted in urine over a 24-hour period to assess overall melatonin production. This method may provide information about the pineal gland's total melatonin output and circadian rhythm.

- Salivary Melatonin Sampling: Saliva samples collected at specific times can be used to measure melatonin levels. Salivary melatonin sampling may be more convenient than blood sampling and can still provide valuable information about melatonin secretion patterns.

- Melatonin Suppression Tests: Melatonin suppression tests involve administering exogenous melatonin or exposing individuals to light to suppress endogenous melatonin secretion. This type of test may be used to evaluate the sensitivity of the pineal gland to light exposure or assess circadian rhythm disorders.

- Imaging Studies: Imaging modalities such as magnetic resonance imaging (MRI) or computed tomography (CT) scans may be used to visualize the pineal gland and detect abnormalities such as tumors or calcifications. Pineal gland tumors (e.g., pinealomas) can affect melatonin secretion and may require medical intervention.

Evaluation of pineal gland function and melatonin secretion may be indicated in individuals with sleep disorders, circadian rhythm disorders, mood disorders, or other conditions associated with altered melatonin levels. Healthcare providers may use a combination of clinical evaluation, laboratory tests, and imaging studies to assess pineal gland health accurately. If you have concerns about your pineal gland function or melatonin levels, it's essential to consult with a healthcare professional for proper evaluation and management.

The thymus gland is an essential part of the immune system, particularly during childhood and adolescence. It plays a crucial role in the development and maturation of T-lymphocytes, a type of white blood cell involved in cell-mediated immunity.

The thymus gland secretes several hormones, such as thyroxin, thymopoietin, and various interleukins, which help regulate immune cell development and function. *Healthcare professionals may assess thymus function and its impact on the immune system through various methods:*

- Thymus Size: The size of the thymus gland can be assessed through imaging studies such as chest X-rays, ultrasound, or magnetic resonance imaging (MRI). Thymus size is typically largest during infancy and childhood, gradually decreasing in size with age. Abnormalities in thymus size or structure may indicate underlying medical conditions such as thymic hyperplasia, thymoma (thymus tumor), or autoimmune diseases affecting the thymus.

- T-Cell Counts: T-lymphocyte counts in the blood can provide information about immune cell function and thymus activity. A decrease in circulating T-cell counts may indicate impaired thymus function or immune deficiency. Conversely, an increase in T-cell counts may occur in response to infections, autoimmune diseases, or other immune-related conditions.

- Hormone Levels: While thymus hormones such as thyroxin are essential for immune function, routine measurement of thymus hormone levels is not typically performed in clinical practice. However, abnormalities in hormone levels may be investigated in specific cases of suspected thymus dysfunction or autoimmune diseases affecting the thymus.

- Immunological Testing: Specialized immunological tests may be performed to assess T-cell function, such as T-cell proliferation assays or cytokine profiling. These tests can provide insights into the immune system's responsiveness and function, which may be influenced by thymus gland activity.

- Thymus Biopsy: In certain cases, a biopsy of the thymus gland may be performed to obtain tissue samples for microscopic examination. Thymus biopsy is typically indicated in the evaluation of suspected thymic tumors, thymic hyperplasia, or autoimmune diseases affecting the thymus.

Assessment of thymus gland function and its impact on the immune system may be indicated in individuals with suspected immune deficiencies, autoimmune diseases, or other immune-related disorders. Healthcare providers may use a combination of clinical evaluation, laboratory tests, imaging studies, and specialized immunological testing to assess thymus health accurately. If you have concerns about your thymus gland function or immune system health, it's essential to consult with a healthcare professional for proper evaluation and management.

Glands throughout the body secrete various hormones and substances that regulate numerous physiological processes. These glands include endocrine glands, which release hormones directly into the bloodstream, as well as exocrine glands, which secrete substances through ducts to specific locations.

Healthcare professionals may assess gland function and hormone levels through various methods:

- Hormone Testing: Hormone levels in the blood or other bodily fluids can be measured to assess gland function. Hormone testing may include assessing levels of thyroid hormones (TSH, T3, T4), adrenal hormones (cortisol, aldosterone), reproductive hormones (estrogen, progesterone, testosterone), pancreatic hormones (insulin, glucagon), and others.

- Imaging Studies: Imaging modalities such as ultrasound, computed tomography (CT), magnetic resonance imaging (MRI), or nuclear medicine scans may be used to visualize glands and detect abnormalities such as tumors, cysts, or structural changes. Imaging studies can help diagnose conditions affecting gland function and hormone production.

- Stimulation and Suppression Tests: These tests involve administering specific substances to stimulate or suppress hormone production by target glands. Examples include the ACTH stimulation test to assess adrenal function, the oral glucose tolerance test to evaluate pancreatic function and insulin secretion, and the TRH stimulation test to assess thyroid function.

Genetic Testing: In some cases, genetic testing may be used to identify inherited disorders affecting gland function. Genetic testing can help diagnose conditions such as familial endocrine neoplasia, congenital adrenal hyperplasia, or inherited thyroid disorders.

Biopsy: A tissue biopsy may be performed to obtain samples from glands for microscopic examination. Biopsy procedures can help diagnose glandular tumors, autoimmune diseases affecting glands, or infections.

Functional Tests: These tests evaluate the functional capacity of glands to perform specific tasks. For example, the sweat test assesses the function of sweat glands in individuals suspected of having cystic fibrosis.

Assessment of gland function and hormone levels may vary depending on the specific glands being evaluated and the suspected underlying conditions. Healthcare providers may use a combination of history taking, physical examination, laboratory tests, imaging studies, and specialized tests to assess gland health and function accurately. If you have concerns about your gland function or hormone levels, it's essential to consult with a healthcare professional for proper evaluation and management.

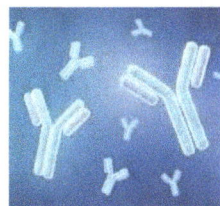

The immunoglobulin index typically refers to a measure of the levels of immunoglobulin in the blood, often used to diagnose and monitor various immune-related disorders. Immunoglobulin, also known as antibodies, are proteins produced by the immune system to help fight off infections and other harmful substances in the body.

There are several types of immunoglobulins, including IgA, IgG, IgM, IgD, and IgE. Each type plays a specific role in the immune response. Abnormal levels of immunoglobulin can indicate various health conditions, such as infections, autoimmune disorders, or immune deficiencies.

The immunoglobulin index may be calculated by comparing the levels of specific immunoglobulin in a patient's blood to normal reference ranges. This comparison helps healthcare providers assess the functioning of the immune system and identify any abnormalities that may require further investigation or treatment.

It's important to consult with a healthcare professional for interpretation of specific immunoglobulin index results, as the significance can vary depending on the individual's medical history and symptoms.

This term **respiratory immune index** could be used colloquially or within a specific research context that I'm not aware of.

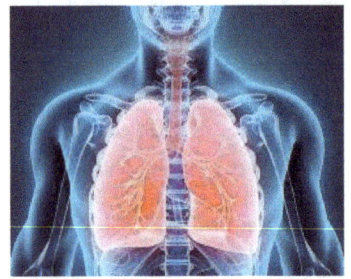

In general, the immune system plays a crucial role in protecting the respiratory tract from infections and other harmful agents. This includes the production of antibodies, activation of immune cells such as macrophages and lymphocytes, and the release of inflammatory mediators in response to pathogens.

There are various markers and indices used in respiratory medicine and immunology to assess the status of the immune system and its response to respiratory infections or diseases. These may include measurements of specific antibodies, cytokine levels, cell counts, or other immunological parameters relevant to respiratory health.

If you encountered the term "respiratory immune index" in a specific context and would like further clarification, providing additional details may help in understanding its meaning or significance. Alternatively, consulting with a healthcare professional or researcher specializing in respiratory medicine or immunology could provide more specific information.

The gastrointestinal (GI) tract is a crucial part of the body's immune system. It is constantly exposed to a variety of pathogens, antigens, and potentially harmful substances from the diet and the environment. Therefore, the immune system in the GI tract plays a vital role in maintaining gut health and preventing infections and inflammation.

In research and clinical settings, various markers and indices may be used to assess the status of the immune system in the gastrointestinal tract. These may include measurements of specific antibodies, cytokine levels, immune cell populations, gut microbiota composition, and other immunological parameters relevant to gastrointestinal health and function.

If you encountered the term "gastrointestinal immune index" in a specific context and would like further clarification, providing additional details may help in understanding its meaning or significance. Consulting with a healthcare professional or researcher specializing in gastroenterology, immunology, or related fields could provide more specific information.

The term "**mucosal immune index**" typically refers to the assessment of the immune system specifically within mucosal surfaces of the body. Mucosal surfaces are found in various parts of the body, including the gastrointestinal tract, respiratory tract, urogenital tract, and ocular surfaces. These surfaces are constantly exposed to potential pathogens and foreign antigens, so the immune system in these areas plays a crucial role in preventing infections while maintaining tolerance to harmless substances like food or commensal bacteria.

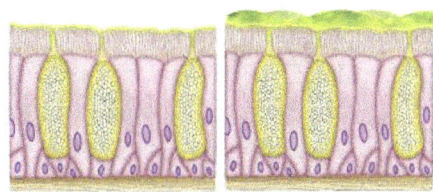

The mucosal immune system differs from the systemic immune system in many ways. It includes specialized immune cells, such as intraepithelial lymphocytes, secretory IgA-producing plasma cells, and mucosa-associated lymphoid tissue (MALT), which are tailored to the unique challenges presented by mucosal surfaces.

Assessing the mucosal immune system may involve various techniques, including:

Measurement of secretory immunoglobulin a (sIgA) levels in mucosal secretions.

Analysis of mucosal immune cell populations using techniques such as flow cytometry or immunohistochemistry.

Evaluation of cytokine levels in mucosal tissues or secretions.

Examination of the integrity and function of mucosal epithelial barriers.

These assessments can provide insights into the immune status of mucosal surfaces, helping to understand immune responses to infections, inflammatory conditions, autoimmune diseases, allergies, and other mucosal disorders.

Studying the mucosal immune index can be particularly relevant in fields such as gastroenterology, respiratory medicine, and immunology, where mucosal surfaces play a significant role in health and disease.

Free thyroxine, often abbreviated as FT4, refers to the unbound, biologically active form of the thyroid hormone thyroxine (T4) circulating in the bloodstream. Thyroxine is produced by the thyroid gland and plays a crucial role in regulating metabolism, growth, and development in the body.

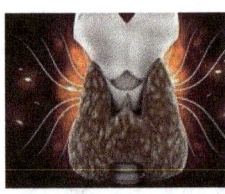

When the thyroid gland produces thyroxine, it releases it into the bloodstream in two forms: bound to proteins (primarily thyroxine-binding globulin, or TBG, as well as albumin and transthyretin) or in its free form. Only the free form of thyroxine is available to tissues and cells to exert its physiological effects. Therefore, measuring the level of free thyroxine is important in assessing thyroid function.

Doctors may order tests to measure free thyroxine levels in the blood to help diagnose thyroid disorders, such as hyperthyroidism (overactive thyroid) or hypothyroidism (underactive thyroid). In hyperthyroidism, free thyroxine levels are typically elevated, while in hypothyroidism, they are usually decreased. Monitoring free thyroxine levels can also help in managing thyroid disorders and adjusting medication doses as needed.

The normal range for free thyroxine levels may vary depending on the laboratory and the specific assay used for testing. It's essential to interpret free thyroxine results in the context of the patient's clinical presentation and other thyroid function tests.

Thyroglobulin is a glycoprotein produced by the thyroid gland. It serves as a precursor in the synthesis of thyroid hormones thyroxine (T4) and triiodothyronine (T3). Thyroglobulin is synthesized by thyroid cells and stored in the follicular lumen of the thyroid gland. When the thyroid gland is stimulated, thyroglobulin is broken down into T4 and T3, which are then released into circulation.

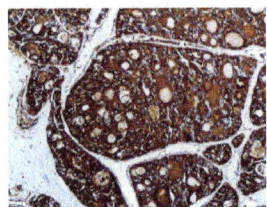

Thyroglobulin is primarily used as a marker in the management of thyroid cancer. After the thyroid gland is surgically removed (thyroidectomy) in individuals with thyroid cancer, thyroglobulin levels should ideally be undetectable or very low. If thyroglobulin levels rise after thyroidectomy, it could indicate the presence of residual thyroid tissue or recurrence of thyroid cancer. Therefore, thyroglobulin levels are monitored regularly, typically in conjunction with thyroid hormone levels and imaging studies, to assess treatment response and detect potential recurrence of thyroid cancer.

In addition to its role in thyroid cancer management, thyroglobulin can also be measured in certain autoimmune thyroid conditions, such as Hashimoto's thyroiditis and Graves' disease, although its clinical utility in these conditions is different from its role in thyroid cancer management.

Thyroglobulin testing is typically done through a blood test, and the results are interpreted in the context of the individual's clinical history and other thyroid function tests.

Anti-thyroglobulin antibodies (also known as anti-TG antibodies) are autoantibodies that target thyroglobulin, a protein produced by the thyroid gland. These antibodies are often found in individuals with autoimmune thyroid diseases, such as Hashimoto's thyroiditis and Graves' disease.

In Hashimoto's thyroiditis, the most common cause of hypothyroidism, the immune system mistakenly attacks the thyroid gland, leading to inflammation and destruction of thyroid tissue. Antithyroglobulin antibodies are often present in the blood of individuals with Hashimoto's thyroiditis, as the immune system targets thyroglobulin, which is abundant in the thyroid gland.

Similarly, in Graves' disease, an autoimmune disorder that causes hyperthyroidism, the immune system produces antibodies that stimulate the thyroid gland to produce excess thyroid hormone. While antithyroglobulin antibodies are less commonly associated with Graves' disease compared to Hashimoto's thyroiditis, they can still be detected in some cases.

Measuring antithyroglobulin antibodies is useful in diagnosing autoimmune thyroid diseases and monitoring their progression. High levels of these antibodies in the blood may indicate autoimmune thyroid disease, even in the absence of symptoms. Monitoring antithyroglobulin antibody levels over time can also help in assessing response to treatment and predicting the risk of future thyroid dysfunction or complications.

It's important to note that while antithyroglobulin antibodies are associated with autoimmune thyroid diseases; their presence alone is not diagnostic of these conditions. The diagnosis is typically made based on a combination of clinical symptoms, physical examination findings, thyroid function tests, imaging studies, and sometimes additional antibody tests.

Triiodothyronine (T3), it is one of the two primary thyroid hormones produced by the thyroid gland, along with thyroxine (T4). T3 is synthesized from T4 in various tissues through the removal of an iodine atom. It plays a crucial role in regulating metabolism, growth, and development in the body.

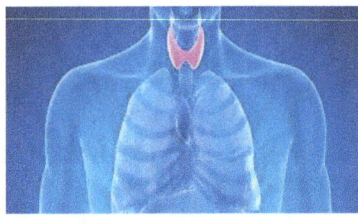

When discussing thyroid function tests, T3 levels are often measured along with other thyroid hormones like T4 and thyroid-stimulating hormone (TSH). Elevated or decreased levels of T3 can indicate thyroid dysfunction, such as hyperthyroidism (elevated T3) or hypothyroidism (decreased T3).

If you meant something else by "three triodothyroinine," please provide more contexts, and I'll be happy to assist you further.

HUMAN TOXIN

A "stimulating beverage" generally refers to a drink that contains substances known to enhance alertness, energy levels, or cognitive function. These beverages often contain stimulants such as caffe ine, which is a central nervous system stimulant found in coffee, tea, energy drinks, and some soft drinks.

Some common stimulating beverages include:

- Coffee: Coffee is one of the most popular stimulating beverages worldwide, known for its caffeine content. It is brewed from roasted coffee beans and can be served hot or cold in various forms, such as espresso, latte, cappuccino, or cold brew.

- Tea: Tea also contains caffeine, albeit in lower amounts compared to coffee. Varieties of tea, such as black tea, green tea, and oolong tea, are made from the leaves of the Camellia sinensis plant and are consumed worldwide for their stimulating and antioxidant properties.

- Energy drinks: Energy drinks are beverages marketed to provide a quick boost in energy and alertness. They typically contain high levels of caffeine, as well as other ingredients such as sugar, taurine, B-vitamins, and herbal extracts like guarana or ginseng.

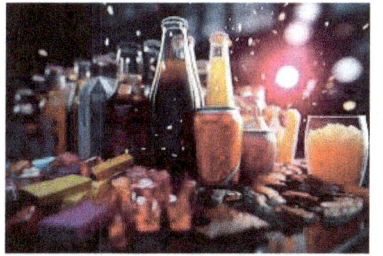

- Soft drinks: Some soft drinks, such as cola beverages, may contain caffeine as an ingredient to provide a mild stimulating effect. However, the caffeine content in soft drinks is generally lower compared to coffee or energy drinks.

- Pre-workout supplements: These are powdered or liquid formulations designed to be consumed before exercise to enhance performance and energy levels. They often contain caffeine, amino acids, vitamins, and other ingredients that promote alertness and improve workout intensity.

While stimulating beverages can provide temporary boosts in energy and alertness, it's essential to consume them in moderation, as excessive intake can lead to negative side effects such as jitteriness, insomnia, increased heart rate, and dependence. Individuals with certain medical conditions or sensitivities to caffeine should also be cautious when consuming stimulating beverages. As always, it's a good idea to consult with a healthcare professional if you have any concerns about your caffeine intake or its effects on your health.

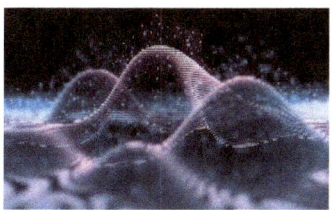

Electromagnetic radiation refers to the propagation of energy through space in the form of electromagnetic waves. These waves consist of oscillating electric and magnetic fields that are perpendicular to each other and to the direction of wave propagation. Electromagnetic radiation encompasses a broad spectrum of wavelengths and frequencies, ranging from extremely low-frequency (ELF) radiation to extremely high-frequency (EHF) radiation.

The electromagnetic spectrum includes various types of radiation, classified based on their wavelengths and frequencies:

- Radio Waves: These have the longest wavelengths and lowest frequencies in the electromagnetic spectrum. They are used for communication, broadcasting, and radar applications.

- Microwaves: Microwaves have shorter wavelengths and higher frequencies than radio waves. They are commonly used in microwave ovens, telecommunications, satellite communications, and radar systems.

- Infrared Radiation (IR): Infrared radiation has wavelengths longer than visible light but shorter than microwaves. It is commonly emitted by warm objects and is used in applications such as thermal imaging, remote sensing, and infrared spectroscopy.

- Visible Light: Visible light is the portion of the electromagnetic spectrum that is visible to the human eye. It includes the colors of the rainbow, ranging from violet (shorter wavelength, higher frequency) to red (longer wavelength, lower frequency).

- Ultraviolet (UV) Radiation: UV radiation has shorter wavelengths and higher frequencies than visible light. It is emitted by the sun and is responsible for suntans, sunburns, and vitamin D synthesis. UV radiation is also used in sterilization, fluorescence, and some medical treatments.

- X-Rays: X-rays have shorter wavelengths and higher frequencies than UV radiation. They have high energy and can penetrate matter, making them useful in medical imaging (X-ray radiography), security screening, and industrial applications.

- Gamma Rays: Gamma rays have the shortest wavelengths and highest frequencies in the electromagnetic spectrum. They are emitted by radioactive substances and nuclear reactions and are used in cancer therapy, sterilization, and scientific research.

Electromagnetic radiation plays a crucial role in various aspects of modern technology, communication, medicine, and scientific research. However, exposure to certain types of electromagnetic radiation, such as UV radiation and X-rays, can pose health risks, including DNA damage, tissue heating, and increased cancer risk. Therefore, it's essential to use protective measures and adhere to safety guidelines when working with or exposed to potentially harmful electromagnetic radiation.

Tobacco and nicotine are closely related substances commonly associated with smoking and other forms of tobacco use. Here's a brief overview of each:

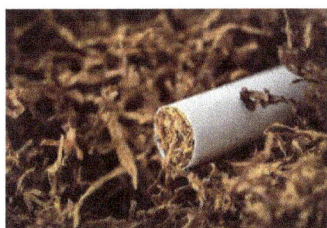

Tobacco: Tobacco refers to the leaves of the Nicotine tobacco and Nicotine rustica plants, which contain nicotine and other compounds. Tobacco has been used for centuries in various forms, including smoking, chewing, and snuffing. When tobacco is smoked, it releases thousands of chemicals, many of which are toxic and carcinogenic. Smoking tobacco is a leading cause of preventable death worldwide, contributing to various health problems such as lung cancer, heart disease, respiratory diseases, and stroke.

Nicotine: Nicotine is a naturally occurring chemical compound found in tobacco plants. It is highly addictive and acts as a stimulant on the central nervous system.

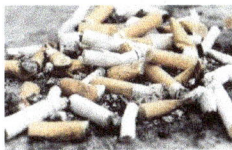

Nicotine is the primary psychoactive ingredient in tobacco products and is responsible for the addictive properties of smoking and other forms of tobacco use. When nicotine is inhaled or absorbed through the skin (as in the case of nicotine patches), it stimulates the release of neurotransmitters such as dopamine, leading to feelings of pleasure and reward. However, repeated exposure to nicotine can lead to tolerance, dependence, and withdrawal symptoms upon cessation.

Despite the known health risks associated with tobacco use, nicotine itself is not considered carcinogenic. However, it is highly addictive, and nicotine addiction is a significant challenge for individuals trying to quit smoking or using other tobacco products. Various nicotine replacement therapies (NRTs), such as nicotine gum, patches, lozenges, and inhalers, are available to help people quit smoking by providing controlled doses of nicotine without the harmful chemicals found in tobacco smoke.

It's important to note that while NRTs can be helpful in managing nicotine withdrawal and facilitating smoking cessation, they are most effective when used as part of a comprehensive quit-smoking program that includes behavioral support and counseling. Additionally, the long-term health effects of using NRTs are generally considered to be much lower than those of continued smoking.

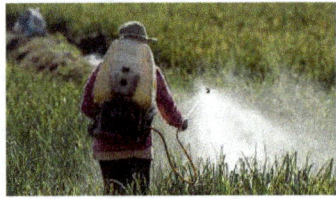

Toxic pesticide residue refers to the presence of harmful chemical residues from pesticides on agricultural products, such as fruits, vegetables, grains, and other crops, after they have been treated with pesticides. Pesticides are chemicals used to control pests, including insects, weeds, and fungi, in order to improve crop yields and prevent economic losses in agriculture.

While pesticides play a crucial role in modern agriculture, their use raises concerns about potential health risks associated with pesticide residues. Some pesticides can persist on food products even after washing or processing, and long-term exposure to these residues has been associated with various health problems, *including:*

- Acute Poisoning: Ingestion or exposure to high levels of certain pesticides can cause acute poisoning, leading to symptoms such as nausea, vomiting, dizziness, headaches, respiratory problems, and, in severe cases, organ damage or death.

- Chronic Health Effects: Chronic exposure to low levels of pesticide residues over time has been linked to an increased risk of certain chronic health conditions, including cancer, neurological disorders, reproductive problems, hormone disruption, and developmental disorders in children.

- Environmental Impact: Pesticide residues can also have adverse effects on the environment, including contamination of soil, water, and air, as well as harm to non-target organisms, such as beneficial insects, birds, and aquatic life.

Regulatory agencies in many countries have established maximum residue limits (MRLs) for pesticides on food products to ensure that they are safe for human consumption. These MRLs are based on scientific risk assessments that take into account factors such as toxicity, exposure levels, and dietary habits. Food producers are required to adhere to these MRLs and follow good agricultural practices to minimize pesticide residues on food.

Consumers can reduce their exposure to pesticide residues by washing fruits and vegetables thoroughly under running water, peeling or trimming outer layers when appropriate, choosing organic produce when possible, and eating a varied diet to minimize exposure to any single pesticide.

It's important for consumers to stay informed about pesticide use in agriculture and advocate for sustainable farming practices that minimize reliance on harmful pesticides while ensuring food safety and environmental protection.

HEAVY METAL

Lead is a naturally occurring element found in the Earth's crust. It has been used by humans for thousands of years due to its versatility, being used in various applications such as construction, plumbing, batteries, ammunition, and paint.

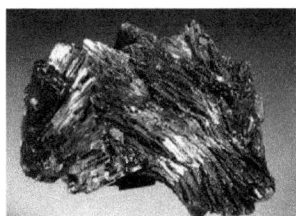

While lead has many useful properties, it is also highly toxic to humans and animals, even in small amounts. Lead exposure can occur through inhalation, ingestion, or absorption through the skin. Once in the body, lead can accumulate in bones, blood, and soft tissues, causing a wide range of adverse health effects, particularly in children and developing fetuses.

Some of the health effects of lead exposure include:

- Neurological Effects: Lead exposure can impair cognitive function, reduce IQ, and cause behavioral problems in children. It can also lead to neurological symptoms such as headaches, memory loss, and nerve damage in adults.

- Developmental Effects: Lead exposure during pregnancy can harm the developing fetus and lead to premature birth, low birth weight, and developmental delays in children.

- Cardiovascular Effects: Lead exposure has been linked to high blood pressure, heart disease, and stroke in adults.

- Kidney Damage: Lead can accumulate in the kidneys and cause kidney damage or failure.

- Reproductive Effects: Lead exposure may affect fertility and reproductive health in both men and women.

- Hematological Effects: Lead exposure can interfere with the production of red blood cells, leading to anemia.

Lead exposure is primarily a concern in environments where lead-based paints, contaminated soil, water pipes, or industrial activities are present. Efforts to reduce lead exposure include regulations to limit lead in consumer products, removal of lead-based paint and pipes, remediation of lead-contaminated sites, and public health education campaigns.

Children and pregnant women are particularly vulnerable to lead exposure, and efforts to prevent childhood lead poisoning are a priority in public health initiatives worldwide. Screening for lead exposure and interventions to reduce exposure are critical to protecting vulnerable populations from the harmful effects of lead.

Mercury is a naturally occurring heavy metal that is found in various forms in the environment. It is present in rocks, soil, water, and the atmosphere. Mercury can also be released into the environment through human activities such as mining, industrial processes, and the burning of fossil fuels.

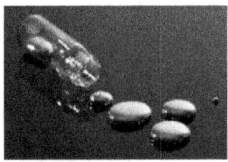 Mercury is a toxic substance that can cause serious health problems in humans and animals. Exposure to mercury can occur through inhalation of mercury vapors, ingestion of contaminated food or water, or absorption through the skin. Once in the body, mercury can accumulate in tissues, particularly in the brain, kidneys, and liver, leading to a range of adverse health effects.

Some of the health effects of mercury exposure include:

- Neurological Effects: Mercury can damage the nervous system, leading to symptoms such as tremors, memory loss, difficulty concentrating, and changes in vision or hearing. Prenatal exposure to mercury can also affect the developing nervous system in fetuses and infants, leading to developmental delays, cognitive impairment, and other neurological problems.

- Cardiovascular Effects: Mercury exposure has been associated with an increased risk of cardiovascular disease, including hypertension, heart attacks, and stroke.

- Renal Effects: Mercury can damage the kidneys, leading to decreased kidney function and renal failure.

- Reproductive Effects: Mercury exposure can affect reproductive health, leading to infertility, miscarriages, and developmental abnormalities in offspring.

- Immune System Effects: Mercury exposure can weaken the immune system, making individuals more susceptible to infections and illnesses.

- Gastrointestinal Effects: Ingestion of mercury can cause gastrointestinal symptoms such as nausea, vomiting, abdominal pain, and diarrhea.

Mercury exists in various forms, including elemental mercury (liquid at room temperature), inorganic mercury compounds, and organic mercury compounds such as methyl mercury. Methyl mercury, which is formed when mercury combines with organic matter in water and soil, is of particular concern due to its ability to bio accumulate in the food chain, especially in predatory fish species.

Efforts to reduce mercury exposure include regulations to limit mercury emissions from industrial sources, measures to reduce mercury use in products such as batteries and thermometers, and advisories to limit consumption of fish known to contain high levels of mercury. Monitoring of mercury levels in the environment and in human populations is also important for assessing and managing the risks associated with mercury exposure.

Cadmium is a naturally occurring metal that is widely distributed in the environment. It is often found in association with zinc, lead, and copper ores, and it is produced as a byproduct of mining and refining these metals. Cadmium is used in various industrial processes, including the production of batteries, pigments, coatings, and plastics. It is also present in some fertilizers and tobacco smoke.

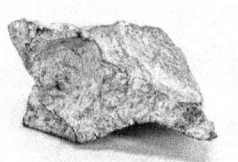

Cadmium is a toxic metal that can pose serious health risks to humans and animals. Exposure to cadmium can occur through inhalation of cadmium-containing dust or fumes, ingestion of contaminated food or water, or absorption through the skin. Once in the body, cadmium accumulates primarily in the kidneys and liver, as well as in bones and other tissues, where it can cause a range of adverse health effects.

Some of the health effects of cadmium exposure include:

- Renal Effects: Cadmium is known to cause kidney damage and may lead to kidney failure with chronic exposure. Cadmium-induced kidney damage is one of the most well-established health effects of cadmium toxicity.

- Bone Effects: Cadmium can replace calcium in bones, leading to a decrease in bone density and an increased risk of osteoporosis and fractures.

- Respiratory Effects: Inhalation of cadmium-containing dust or fumes can irritate the respiratory tract and cause symptoms such as coughing, wheezing, and shortness of breath. Long-term exposure may also increase the risk of lung cancer.

- Cardiovascular Effects: Cadmium exposure has been associated with an increased risk of cardiovascular disease, including hypertension, heart attacks, and stroke.

- Reproductive Effects: Cadmium exposure may affect reproductive health, leading to decreased fertility, miscarriages, and developmental abnormalities in offspring.

- Cancer: Cadmium is classified as a known human carcinogen by the International Agency for Research on Cancer (IARC). Long-term exposure to cadmium has been linked to an increased risk of lung, prostate, and kidney cancers.

Efforts to reduce cadmium exposure include regulations to limit cadmium emissions from industrial sources, measures to minimize occupational exposure in workplaces where cadmium is used or produced, and advisories to limit consumption of cadmium-contaminated foods such as shellfish and certain grains. Monitoring of cadmium levels in the environment and in human populations is also important for assessing and managing the risks associated with cadmium exposure.

Chromium is a naturally occurring transition metal found in the Earth's crust. It exists in various oxidation states, with chromium (III) and chromium (VI) being the most common forms. Chromium (III) is an essential nutrient required in trace amounts for human health, playing a role in glucose metabolism and insulin action.

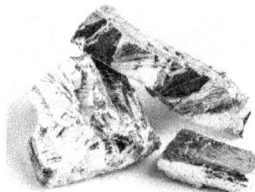

However, chromium (VI), also known as hexavalent chromium, is highly toxic and poses significant health risks to humans and the environment. Hexavalent chromium compounds are often produced by industrial processes, such as chrome plating, stainless steel production, leather tanning, and pigment manufacturing.

It is also a byproduct of certain industrial activities like welding and thermal cutting of stainless steel.

Exposure to hexavalent chromium can occur through inhalation of dust or fumes, ingestion of contaminated food or water, or contact with contaminated soil or water. Once in the body, hexavalent chromium can cause a range of adverse health effects, *including:*

- Respiratory Effects: Inhalation of hexavalent chromium compounds can irritate the respiratory tract and cause symptoms such as coughing, wheezing, and shortness of breath. Chronic exposure may increase the risk of lung cancer and respiratory diseases such as bronchitis and asthma.

- Dermal Effects: Contact with hexavalent chromium compounds can cause skin irritation, dermatitis, and allergic reactions. Prolonged or repeated exposure may lead to ulceration and skin sensitization.

- Gastrointestinal Effects: Ingestion of hexavalent chromium can irritate the gastrointestinal tract and cause symptoms such as nausea, vomiting, abdominal pain, and diarrhea.

- Carcinogenicity: Hexavalent chromium is classified as a known human carcinogen by the International Agency for Research on Cancer (IARC). Long-term exposure to hexavalent chromium compounds has been linked to an increased risk of lung cancer, nasal cancer, and other cancers.

Efforts to reduce hexavalent chromium exposure include regulations to limit emissions from industrial sources, implementation of engineering controls and personal protective equipment in workplaces where hexavalent chromium is used, and remediation of contaminated sites. Monitoring of hexavalent chromium levels in the environment and in human populations is also important for assessing and managing the risks associated with exposure.

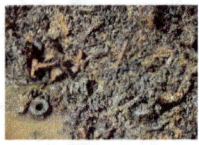

Arsenic is a naturally occurring element found in the Earth's crust. It is widely distributed in the environment and can be present in soil, water, air, and food. Arsenic exists in various forms, including inorganic arsenic compounds (such as arsenite and arsenate) and organic arsenic compounds. Inorganic arsenic is generally considered more toxic than organic arsenic.

Exposure to arsenic can occur through various pathways, including ingestion of contaminated water or food, inhalation of airborne arsenic particles, and dermal contact with arsenic-containing substances. Arsenic contamination in drinking water is a significant public health concern in many parts of the world, particularly in regions where natural geological sources contain high levels of arsenic.

Arsenic is a potent toxicant that can cause a range of adverse health effects in humans, including:

- Acute Poisoning: Ingestion of high levels of arsenic can cause acute poisoning, leading to symptoms such as nausea, vomiting, abdominal pain, diarrhea, and, in severe cases, shock, coma, and death.

- Chronic Health Effects: Chronic exposure to lower levels of arsenic over time can lead to a variety of long-term health problems, including skin lesions (such as hyperpigmentation and keratosis), peripheral neuropathy, cardiovascular disease, respiratory issues, diabetes, and various types of cancer, including skin, lung, bladder, and kidney cancer. Chronic arsenic exposure has also been associated with developmental and reproductive effects, including reduced fetal growth and increased risk of miscarriage.

Arsenic toxicity depends on factors such as the chemical form of arsenic, the route and duration of exposure, and individual susceptibility factors such as age, genetics, and overall health status. The World Health Organization (WHO) and other regulatory agencies have established guidelines and standards for arsenic levels in drinking water and food to protect public health.

Efforts to mitigate arsenic exposure include the implementation of water treatment technologies to remove arsenic from drinking water sources, remediation of contaminated sites, regulation of arsenic levels in food and consumer products, and public health education and outreach to raise awareness about the risks of arsenic exposure and methods for reducing exposure. Regular monitoring of arsenic levels in environmental media and biological samples is also essential for assessing and managing the risks associated with arsenic exposure.

Antimony is a chemical element with the symbol Sb and atomic number 51. It is a silvery-white, brittle, semi-metallic element that occurs naturally in the Earth's crust. Antimony is primarily obtained from the mineral stibnite (antimony sulfide), but it is also found in other minerals.

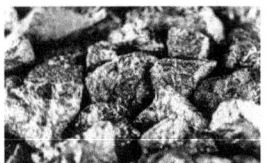

Antimony has various industrial applications due to its unique properties. *Some common uses of antimony include:*

- Alloys: Antimony is often used as an alloying element in combination with other metals, such as lead, to improve their mechanical properties. Lead-antimony alloys are commonly used in batteries, ammunition, solder, and bearings.

- Flame Retardants: Antimony compounds are used as flame retardants in plastics, textiles, and other materials to reduce the risk of fire and slow down the spread of flames.

- Catalysts: Antimony compounds are used as catalysts in the production of polyester fibers and polyethylene terephthalate (PET) plastics.

- Glass and Ceramics: Antimony trioxide (Sb_2O_3) is used as a fining agent in the production of glass and ceramics to improve clarity and strength.

- Medicine: Antimony compounds have been used in traditional medicine for their supposed medicinal properties, although their use in modern medicine is limited due to their toxicity.

Despite its industrial importance, antimony can be toxic to humans and animals, particularly in its inorganic forms. Chronic exposure to antimony compounds has been associated with a range of health effects, including respiratory problems, skin irritation, gastrointestinal symptoms, cardiovascular effects, and reproductive and developmental toxicity. Antimony exposure can occur through inhalation of airborne particles, ingestion of contaminated food or water, or dermal contact with antimony-containing substances.

Regulatory agencies such as the U.S. Environmental Protection Agency (EPA) have established guidelines and standards for antimony levels in drinking water and occupational settings to protect public health. Efforts to mitigate antimony exposure include the use of engineering controls and personal protective equipment in workplaces where antimony is used, regulation of antimony levels in consumer products, and public health education and outreach to raise awareness about the risks of antimony exposure and methods for reducing exposure.

Thallium is a chemical element with the symbol Tl and atomic number 81. It is a soft, bluish-white metal that is highly toxic, with no known biological function in humans. Thallium compounds were historically used in various industrial and commercial applications, but due to their extreme toxicity, many of these uses have been discontinued or strictly regulated.

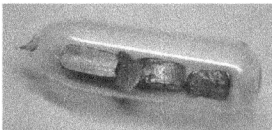

Thallium poisoning can occur through ingestion, inhalation, or dermal contact with thallium compounds. Once in the body, thallium can interfere with various cellular processes, disrupt enzyme function, and cause severe damage to multiple organ systems. Thallium poisoning can lead to a wide range of symptoms, depending on the level and duration of exposure, including:

Gastrointestinal Symptoms: Nausea, vomiting, abdominal pain, and diarrhea are common gastrointestinal symptoms of thallium poisoning.

Neurological Symptoms: Thallium toxicity affects the nervous system, leading to symptoms such as headache, dizziness, confusion, seizures, tremors, and sensory disturbances (such as numbness, tingling, or burning sensations in the extremities).

- Cardiovascular Symptoms: Thallium poisoning can cause abnormalities in heart rate and rhythm, leading to chest pain, palpitations, and potentially life-threatening cardiac arrhythmias.

- Dermatological Symptoms: Skin changes, such as hair loss (alopecia), hyperpigmentation, and rash, are common dermatological manifestations of thallium poisoning.

- Renal and Hepatic Dysfunction: Thallium toxicity can lead to kidney and liver damage, resulting in impaired renal function and liver failure.

Thallium poisoning is a medical emergency that requires prompt diagnosis and treatment. Treatment may include supportive measures to manage symptoms, chelation therapy to remove thallium from the body, and supportive care to address complications such as dehydration, electrolyte imbalances, and organ failure.

Due to its high toxicity and potential for misuse as a poison, thallium compounds are strictly regulated in many countries. Efforts to mitigate thallium exposure include restrictions on the use of thallium in consumer products and industrial processes, occupational safety measures to minimize exposure in workplaces where thallium is used, and public health education and outreach to raise awareness about the risks of thallium exposure and methods for preventing poisoning.

Aluminum, also spelled aluminum in some regions, is a chemical element with the symbol Al and atomic number 13. It is a silvery-white, lightweight metal that is the third most abundant element in the Earth's crust, after oxygen and silicon. Aluminum is highly reactive and is rarely found in its pure form in nature; instead, it is typically found in various minerals such as bauxite, cryolite, and feldspar.

Aluminum has numerous industrial, commercial, and technological applications due to its unique properties, *which include:*

- Lightweight: Aluminum is lightweight and has a low density, making it ideal for use in applications where weight reduction is important, such as aerospace, automotive, and transportation industries.

- Corrosion Resistance: Aluminum forms a thin, protective oxide layer on its surface that provides excellent corrosion resistance, making it suitable for outdoor and marine applications, as well as in the construction of structures and buildings.

- Conductivity: Aluminum is an excellent conductor of electricity and heat, making it useful in electrical transmission lines, heat exchangers, and electronic devices.

- Malleability and Ductility: Aluminum is highly malleable and ductile, allowing it to be easily formed into various shapes and structures using common manufacturing processes such as rolling, extrusion, and forging.

- Reflectivity: Aluminum has high reflectivity for both visible light and thermal radiation, making it useful in applications such as reflective coatings, mirrors, and solar panels.

Some common uses of aluminum include:

- Transportation: Aluminum is used in the construction of aircraft, automobiles, trains, and bicycles due to its lightweight and strength-to-weight ratio.
- Packaging: Aluminum is widely used in packaging materials such as beverage cans, food containers, foil wraps, and aerosol cans.

- Construction: Aluminum is used in the construction industry for building facades, window frames, roofing, cladding, and structural components.

- Electrical and Electronics: Aluminum is used in electrical transmission lines, heat sinks, capacitors, and electronic enclosures.

- Consumer Goods: Aluminum is used in a wide range of consumer products such as cookware, utensils, furniture, appliances, and sporting goods.

While aluminum is generally considered safe for most applications, there has been some concern about potential health risks associated with aluminum exposure, particularly in relation to food and beverage packaging, antiperspirants, and aluminum-containing medications. However, regulatory agencies such as the U.S. Food and Drug Administration (FDA) and the European Food Safety Authority (EFSA) have determined that aluminum exposure from these sources is typically low and does not pose a significant health risk for most people.

BASIC PHYSICAL QUALITY

"**Response ability**" is a term that combines "response" and "ability" and refers to the capacity or capability to respond effectively to a given situation or circumstance. It encompasses the skills, resources, knowledge, and attributes needed to address challenges, solve problems, and adapt to changing circumstances.

Having response ability involves several key elements:

Awareness: Being aware of one's surroundings, circumstances, and the needs of others is essential for effective response ability. This includes understanding the context and implications of a situation and recognizing the potential consequences of different actions.

- Adaptability: Response ability often requires the ability to adapt to changing conditions and unforeseen challenges. This may involve being flexible, creative, and open to new ideas and approaches.

- Resilience: Building resilience is important for response ability, as it enables individuals to bounce back from setbacks, overcome obstacles, and persevere in the face of adversity.

- Problem-solving: Having strong problem-solving skills is crucial for response ability. This involves identifying issues, analyzing root causes, generating solutions, and implementing effective strategies to address them.

- Communication: Effective communication is essential for response ability, as it enables individuals to convey information, coordinate actions, and collaborate with others to achieve common goals.

- Empathy: Response ability also involves empathy, or the ability to understand and share the feelings of others. This helps individuals respond to the needs of others in a compassionate and empathetic manner.

Overall, response ability is about being proactive, resourceful, and responsible in addressing challenges and opportunities. It is a fundamental skill that is valuable in both personal and professional contexts, as it enables individuals to navigate complex situations, build positive relationships, and achieve meaningful outcomes.

"Mental power" typically refers to the cognitive abilities and capacities of the mind, including aspects such as intelligence, memory, concentration, creativity, problem-solving skills, and emotional intelligence. It encompasses the mental faculties that enable individuals to think, learn, reason, perceive, remember, and adapt to their environment.

Here are some key components of mental power:

- Intelligence: Intelligence refers to the ability to understand complex ideas, learn from experience, adapt to new situations, and solve problems effectively. It encompasses various cognitive abilities, including reasoning, critical thinking, and abstract thinking.

- Memory: Memory is the ability to encode, store, and retrieve information. It plays a crucial role in learning, decision-making, and everyday functioning. Different types of memory include short-term memory, long-term memory, and working memory.

- Concentration and Focus: Concentration and focus refer to the ability to sustain attention on a task or stimulus for an extended period. Strong concentration skills are essential for learning, productivity, and achieving goals.

- Creativity: Creativity involves the ability to generate novel ideas, solutions, and insights. It encompasses thinking outside the box, making connections between seemingly unrelated concepts, and approaching problems from different perspectives.

- Problem-solving Skills: Problem-solving skills involve the ability to identify, analyze, and solve problems effectively. This includes breaking down complex problems into manageable components, generating alternative solutions, and evaluating their effectiveness.

- Emotional Intelligence: Emotional intelligence refers to the ability to recognize, understand, and manage one's own emotions, as well as the emotions of others. It involves skills such as self-awareness, self-regulation, empathy, and social skills.

- Critical Thinking: Critical thinking involves the ability to analyze, evaluate, and interpret information objectively and logically. It includes skills such as reasoning, analysis, interpretation, inference, and evaluation.

Developing and enhancing mental power requires practice, effort, and continuous learning. Strategies for improving mental power include engaging in activities that challenge the mind, such as puzzles, reading, learning new skills, practicing mindfulness and meditation, seeking feedback, and pursuing personal development goals. Additionally, maintaining a healthy lifestyle, including regular exercise, adequate sleep, and a balanced diet, can support cognitive function and mental well-being.

Water shortage, also known as dehydration, occurs when there is an inadequate intake or excessive loss of water from the body, leading to an imbalance in the body's fluid levels. The human body requires water for various essential functions, including regulating body temperature, transporting nutrients and oxygen to cells, flushing out waste products, and lubricating joints.

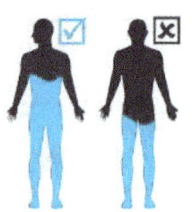

When the body loses more water than it takes in, dehydration can occur, resulting in a range of symptoms and health effects. Some common signs and symptoms of dehydration include:

- Thirst: Thirst is the body's natural mechanism for signaling the need for water. Feeling thirsty is often one of the first signs of dehydration.

- Dry Mouth and Lips: Dehydration can cause dryness in the mouth and lips due to decreased saliva production.

- Dark Urine: Urine color can be a useful indicator of hydration status. Dark yellow or amber-colored urine may indicate dehydration, while pale yellow or clear urine is a sign of adequate hydration.

- Decreased Urination: Reduced urine output or infrequent urination may occur with dehydration as the body conserves water.

- Fatigue and Weakness: Dehydration can lead to feelings of fatigue, weakness, and lethargy, as the body's cells may not function optimally without adequate hydration.

- Dizziness and Lightheadedness: Dehydration can cause dizziness, lightheadedness, and fainting due to decreased blood volume and blood pressure.

- Headache: Dehydration may contribute to headaches and migraines, as reduced fluid levels can affect blood flow and oxygen delivery to the brain.

- Dry Skin: Inadequate hydration can lead to dry, flaky skin and an increased risk of skin problems such as eczema and dermatitis.

- Muscle Cramps: Dehydration may result in muscle cramps, spasms, and weakness, as electrolyte imbalances can affect muscle function.

- Confusion and Irritability: Severe dehydration can impair cognitive function, leading to confusion, irritability, and difficulty concentrating.

In severe cases, dehydration can lead to serious complications, including heat exhaustion, heatstroke, kidney failure, and even death if left untreated. It is essential to drink water regularly throughout the day and stay hydrated, especially during hot weather, physical activity, illness, or other situations that increase fluid loss. Maintaining a balanced diet rich in hydrating foods such as fruits and vegetables can also help prevent dehydration. If dehydration is suspected, it is important to seek medical attention promptly, particularly for severe or persistent symptoms.

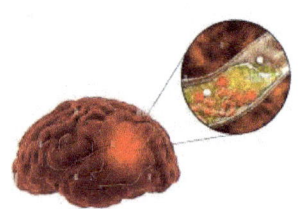

Hypoxia is a medical condition characterized by a deficiency in the amount of oxygen reaching the body's tissues and organs. Oxygen is essential for cellular metabolism and energy production, and when oxygen levels are insufficient, cells may not function properly, leading to a range of adverse effects.

There are several types of hypoxia, each with different causes and manifestations:

- Hypoxic Hypoxia: This type of hypoxia occurs when there is a decrease in the partial pressure of oxygen in the blood, leading to inadequate oxygenation of tissues. Causes of hypoxic hypoxia include high altitudes, where the air pressure and oxygen levels are lower, as well as conditions that impair the lungs' ability to absorb oxygen, such as pneumonia, pulmonary edema, or respiratory failure.

- Anemic Hypoxia: Anemic hypoxia occurs when the blood is unable to carry enough oxygen due to a decrease in the concentration of hemoglobin or a decrease in the oxygen-carrying capacity of hemoglobin. Causes of anemic hypoxia include anemia (low red blood cell count), hemoglobinopathies (such as sickle cell disease), and carbon monoxide poisoning, which can bind to hemoglobin and reduce its ability to carry oxygen.

- Ischemic Hypoxia: Ischemic hypoxia occurs when there is inadequate blood flow to tissues, leading to reduced oxygen delivery. Causes of ischemic hypoxia include cardiovascular conditions such as heart failure, shock, or circulatory shock, which can impair blood flow to organs and tissues.

- Histotoxic Hypoxia: Histotoxic hypoxia occurs when cells are unable to use oxygen effectively due to the presence of toxins or metabolic inhibitors. Causes of histotoxic hypoxia include exposure to certain drugs or chemicals that interfere with cellular respiration, such as cyanide.

Symptoms of hypoxia can vary depending on the severity and duration of oxygen deprivation, as well as the affected organs and tissues. *Common symptoms of hypoxia include:*

- Shortness of breath
- Rapid breathing (hyperventilation)
- Cyanosis (bluish discoloration of the skin, lips, or nail beds)
- Confusion or disorientation
- Headache
- Dizziness or lightheadedness
- Rapid heart rate (tachycardia)
- Fatigue or weakness
- Nausea or vomiting
- Loss of consciousness

Hypoxia is a serious medical emergency that requires prompt evaluation and treatment to prevent complications and restore adequate oxygenation to the tissues. Treatment of hypoxia may involve supplemental oxygen therapy, addressing the underlying cause of oxygen deprivation, and supportive measures to stabilize the patient's condition. In severe cases, interventions such as mechanical ventilation or administration of medications to improve cardiac function may be necessary.

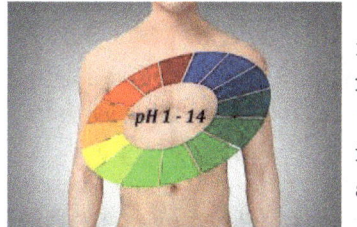

The pH of the human body refers to the measurement of the acidity or alkalinity of bodily fluids and tissues. pH is a scale ranging from 0 to 14, with 7 considered neutral. Values below 7 indicate acidity, while values above 7 indicate alkalinity.

Different parts of the human body have varying pH levels, which are tightly regulated to maintain homeostasis and support proper physiological function. *Here are some examples of pH levels in different parts of the body:*

- Blood: The pH of arterial blood is typically maintained within a narrow range of 7.35 to 7.45. Values below this range (acidosis) or above this range

(alkalosis) can indicate metabolic or respiratory disturbances and can have serious health implications.
- Stomach: The stomach has an acidic environment to aid in the digestion of food. Gastric acid, composed mainly of hydrochloric acid (HCl), gives the stomach a pH ranging from approximately 1.5 to 3.5.

- Urine: The pH of urine can vary depending on factors such as diet, hydration status, and underlying health conditions. The normal pH range for urine is typically between 4.5 and 8.0, with values below 7 being acidic and values above 7 being alkaline.
- Skin: The skin's pH is slightly acidic, with a typical range of 4.5 to 5.5. This acidity helps to protect the skin from harmful microorganisms and maintain the integrity of the skin barrier.

- Saliva: Saliva has a pH ranging from approximately 6.2 to 7.6, with an average pH around 6.7. Saliva helps to neutralize acids in the mouth, maintain oral health, and facilitate digestion.

- Intestines: The pH of the small intestine is slightly alkaline, ranging from approximately 7.0 to 8.5. This alkalinity supports the activity of digestive enzymes and promotes nutrient absorption. The pH of the large intestine is slightly more acidic, typically ranging from 5.5 to 7.0.

The body's ability to regulate pH is essential for maintaining cellular function, enzyme activity, and overall health. Various physiological mechanisms, such as the bicarbonate buffer system, respiratory regulation of carbon dioxide levels, and renal excretion of acids and bases, help to maintain pH homeostasis despite changes in internal and external conditions. Imbalances in pH can disrupt normal physiological processes and contribute to health problems, so maintaining proper pH balance is critical for overall well-being.

ALLERGY

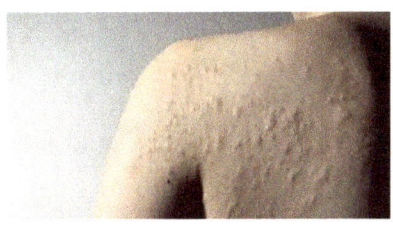
The term **"drug allergy index"** typically refers to a system or tool used to assess the likelihood or severity of an allergic reaction to a specific drug or class of drugs. Allergic reactions to medications can range from mild skin rashes to life-threatening anaphylaxis and can occur with any medication, including over-the-counter drugs, prescription medications, and herbal supplements.

Several factors may contribute to the risk of developing a drug allergy, including:

- Previous Allergic Reactions: Individuals with a history of allergic reactions to specific medications or drug classes are at increased risk of developing allergies to those drugs in the future.

- Drug Characteristics: Some drugs are more likely to cause allergic reactions due to their chemical structure, metabolism, or mechanisms of action.

- Genetic Factors: Genetic predisposition may play a role in determining an individual's susceptibility to drug allergies.
- Underlying Health Conditions: Certain medical conditions, such as asthma, allergic rhinitis, or autoimmune diseases, may increase the risk of developing drug allergies.

- Immunological Factors: Allergic reactions to medications typically involve an immune response mediated by antibodies, such as immunoglobulin E (IgE), or other immune cells.

A drug allergy index may take into account various factors to estimate the risk of allergic reactions to specific drugs or drug classes. This index could include information such as:

- Patient History: Previous allergic reactions to medications, including type and severity of reaction.
- Drug Characteristics: Chemical structure, pharmacological properties, and known allergenic potential of the drug.

- Cross-Reactivity: Potential for cross-reactivity with other drugs or substances due to shared structural features.

- Underlying Risk Factors: Presence of underlying health conditions or genetic factors that may increase susceptibility to drug allergies.

- Immunological Markers: Laboratory tests, such as skin prick testing or measurement of specific IgE antibodies, to assess allergic sensitization.

The goal of a drug allergy index is to help healthcare providers make informed decisions about drug prescribing, minimize the risk of allergic reactions, and provide appropriate management for patients with known or suspected drug allergies. However, it's important to note that drug allergies can be complex and unpredictable, and not all allergic reactions can be accurately predicted based on risk assessment tools. Therefore, healthcare providers must carefully evaluate each patient's individual risk factors and medical history when prescribing medications.

While alcohol intolerance or sensitivity is relatively common, true **alcohol allergies** are rare. An alcohol allergy index doesn't exist in the same way that indices for other allergies might, mainly because true alcohol allergies are not as prevalent or well-defined as allergies to other substances like foods, medications, or environmental allergens.

However, some factors could contribute to the likelihood or severity of an adverse reaction to alcohol:

- Genetic Predisposition: Some individuals may have genetic factors that predispose them to adverse reactions to alcohol, such as deficiencies in enzymes involved in alcohol metabolism.

- Underlying Conditions: Certain medical conditions, such as asthma, hay fever, or allergic rhinitis, may increase the risk of developing an adverse reaction to alcohol.

- Histamine Sensitivity: Alcohol, particularly in certain beverages like wine and beer, can contain histamine, which may trigger allergic-like symptoms in individuals sensitive to histamine.

- Sulfite Sensitivity: Some alcoholic beverages, particularly wines, may contain sulfites, which can cause adverse reactions in individuals sensitive to sulfites.

- Additives and Preservatives: Alcoholic beverages may contain additives or preservatives that could trigger allergic reactions in susceptible individuals.

- Cross-Reactivity: Individuals with known allergies to certain foods or substances may experience cross-reactivity with components in alcoholic beverages, leading to allergic-like symptoms.

Symptoms of adverse reactions to alcohol can vary widely and may include:

- Flushing or redness of the skin (especially in the face)
- Hives or skin rash
- Itching or tingling sensation in the mouth or throat
- Nasal congestion or runny nose
- Headache
- Nausea or vomiting
- Difficulty breathing
- Rapid heartbeat
- Drop in blood pressure

If someone suspects they may have an allergy or intolerance to alcohol, they should consult with a healthcare professional for proper evaluation and diagnosis. Testing for alcohol allergies may involve skin prick tests or blood tests to measure specific IgE antibodies. In cases of severe reactions or anaphylaxis, it's crucial to seek immediate medical attention.

Overall, while true alcohol allergies are rare, individuals who experience adverse reactions to alcohol should avoid consuming it and consult with a healthcare provider for appropriate management and guidance.

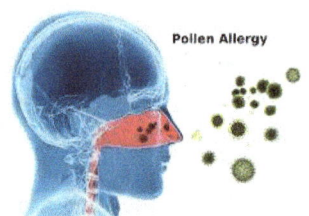
A pollen allergy index, also known as a pollen count or pollen forecast, is a tool used to measure and predict the levels of pollen in the air. This information helps individuals with pollen allergies (also known as hay fever or allergic rhinitis) anticipate and manage their symptoms. Pollen allergy indices are typically provided by weather agencies, environmental organizations, or allergy research institutions.

Here's how a pollen allergy index typically works:

- Measurement of Pollen Levels: Pollen counts are measured by collecting air samples using specialized equipment, such as pollen traps or volumetric samplers. These samples are then analyzed under a microscope to identify and count the different types of pollen grains present.

- Classification of Pollen Levels: Pollen levels are usually classified into categories based on the concentration of pollen grains in the air. Common categories include low, moderate, high, and very high pollen levels. Some indices may also provide specific information about the types of pollen grains that are most prevalent.

- Forecasting: Pollen allergy indices often include forecasts that predict pollen levels for upcoming days or weeks. These forecasts take into account factors such as weather conditions, seasonal patterns, and historical pollen data.

- Presentation of Information: Pollen allergy indices are typically presented in the form of charts, graphs, or maps that show pollen levels over time or across different geographic regions. This information may be available through websites, mobile apps, or news broadcasts.

- Guidance for Allergy Management: Pollen allergy indices may also include recommendations and tips for managing allergy symptoms during periods of high pollen levels. This may include advice on avoiding outdoor activities, keeping windows closed, using air purifiers or pollen filters, and taking allergy medications as needed.

The purpose of a pollen allergy index is to help individuals with pollen allergies plan their activities and take appropriate precautions to minimize exposure to pollen during times when levels are high. By staying informed about pollen levels and taking proactive steps to manage symptoms, allergy sufferers can reduce their discomfort and maintain their quality of life, even during allergy seasons.

Allergic reactions to injections can occur due to various reasons, *including:*

- Medication Components: Some individuals may be allergic to certain components of injected medications, such as preservatives, stabilizers, or inactive ingredients.

- Latex Allergy: Latex allergy is a common type of allergy that can be triggered by exposure to latex-containing medical products, including syringes, gloves, or injection site materials.

- Medication Allergies: Allergic reactions can occur in response to the active ingredient(s) in a medication administered via injection.

- Adverse Reactions: Not all reactions to injections are true allergic reactions. Some reactions may be non-allergic, such as irritation at the injection site or side effects related to the medication's pharmacological action.

If someone experiences an allergic reaction to an injection, it's essential to assess the severity of the reaction and determine its cause. *Common symptoms of allergic reactions to injections include:*

- Itching or hives at the injection site
- Swelling or redness at the injection site
- Difficulty breathing or wheezing
- Rapid heartbeat
- Drop in blood pressure
- Nausea or vomiting
- Dizziness or fainting
- Anaphylaxis (a severe, life-threatening allergic reaction)

➤ Management of injection allergies typically involves:

- Immediate Treatment: In cases of severe allergic reactions or anaphylaxis, prompt administration of epinephrine (adrenaline) and emergency medical care are necessary.

- Identifying the Allergen: Determining the specific cause of the allergic reaction through diagnostic tests, such as skin prick tests or blood tests, can help identify the allergen(s) responsible for the reaction.

- Avoidance: Once the allergen is identified, efforts should be made to avoid exposure to it in the future. This may involve using alternative medications or medical products that do not contain the allergen.

- Desensitization: In some cases, allergen immunotherapy or desensitization may be considered as a treatment option to reduce allergic reactions over time.

If someone suspects they have experienced an allergic reaction to an injection, they should seek immediate medical attention for evaluation and appropriate management. Allergy evaluation and management should be conducted under the guidance of a qualified healthcare professional, such as an allergist or immunologist.

An **"allergy index"** for chemical products is not a standardized concept in the same way as indices for pollen or other environmental allergens. However, it's essential to understand how individuals may develop allergic reactions to various chemical products and how these reactions can be managed.

Chemical products can contain a wide range of substances that have the potential to trigger allergic reactions in susceptible individuals. Common sources of chemical allergies include:

Cosmetics and Personal Care Products: Ingredients commonly found in cosmetics, skincare products, hair dyes, and fragrances can cause allergic reactions in some individuals. These may include preservatives, fragrances, dyes, and other additives.

- Cleaning Products: Household cleaning products, such as detergents, disinfectants, and surface cleaners, can contain irritants or allergens that may cause skin or respiratory reactions.

- Latex: Latex allergy can be triggered by exposure to natural rubber latex, which is found in many medical and non-medical products, including gloves, condoms, balloons, and rubber bands.

- Medications: Some medications, particularly topical medications or those administered via injection, can contain allergenic ingredients that may cause allergic reactions in susceptible individuals.

- Industrial Chemicals: Workers in industries such as construction, manufacturing, and agriculture may be exposed to various industrial chemicals that can cause allergic contact dermatitis or respiratory sensitization.

- Household Products: Other household items, such as adhesives, paints, solvents, and pesticides, can contain chemicals that may trigger allergic reactions or irritate the skin or respiratory system.

Symptoms of allergic reactions to chemical products can vary depending on the type of allergen and the route of exposure. *Common symptoms may include:*

- Skin reactions, such as redness, itching, rash, or hives
- Respiratory symptoms, such as sneezing, coughing, wheezing, or shortness of breath
- Eye irritation or inflammation
- Nasal congestion or runny nose
- Headache or dizziness
- Nausea or vomiting

Management of chemical allergies involves:

- Avoidance: Identifying and avoiding exposure to the allergen(s) responsible for the allergic reaction is the primary strategy for managing chemical allergies. This may involve reading product labels, choosing alternative products, or using personal protective equipment to minimize exposure.

- Symptom Relief: Over-the-counter medications, such as antihistamines or corticosteroid creams, may help alleviate symptoms of allergic reactions. In severe cases, prescription medications or medical intervention may be necessary.

- Allergy Testing: Allergy testing, such as patch testing or skin prick testing, may be recommended to identify specific allergens responsible for allergic reactions.

- Education and Awareness: Educating individuals about common allergens and strategies for avoiding exposure can help prevent allergic reactions and improve overall quality of life.

If someone suspects they have experienced an allergic reaction to a chemical product, they should seek medical attention for evaluation and appropriate management. Allergy evaluation and management should be conducted under the guidance of a qualified healthcare professional, such as an allergist or dermatologist.

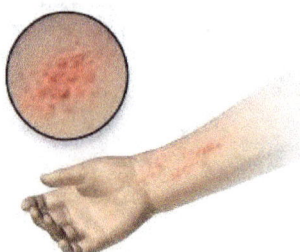

A "**paint allergy index**" isn't a standardized term, but it can be understood as a measure of the likelihood or severity of allergic reactions to paint or paint-related products. Allergic reactions to paint can occur due to exposure to various components found in paints, such as solvents, pigments, preservatives, and other additives.

Symptoms of allergic reactions to paint can vary widely and may include:

- ➤ Skin irritation or rash (contact dermatitis) at the site of contact with paint
- ➤ Redness, swelling, or blistering of the skin
- ➤ Itching or hives
- ➤ Respiratory symptoms, such as coughing, wheezing, or shortness of breath

- Nasal congestion or runny nose
- Eye irritation or inflammation
- Headache or dizziness

It's important to note that not all reactions to paint are allergic in nature. Some individuals may experience non-allergic reactions, such as irritation or sensitivity, to paint fumes or components.

Several factors may contribute to the risk of developing allergic reactions to paint:

- Sensitizing Agents: Certain chemicals found in paints, such as formaldehyde, volatile organic compounds (VOCs), and acrylic resins, can act as sensitizing agents and trigger allergic reactions in susceptible individuals.

- Previous Exposure: Individuals who have been previously exposed to paint or paint-related products may develop sensitivities or allergies over time.

- Occupational Exposure: Workers in industries such as painting, construction, or renovation may be at increased risk of developing allergic reactions to paint due to repeated or prolonged exposure.
- Pre-existing Allergies: Individuals with pre-existing allergies or respiratory conditions, such as asthma or allergic rhinitis, may be more susceptible to developing allergic reactions to paint.

Management of paint allergies involves:

- Avoiding exposure to paints or paint-related products that trigger allergic reactions
- Using personal protective equipment, such as gloves, masks, or goggles, when working with paints
- Ensuring adequate ventilation in indoor spaces to minimize exposure to paint fumes
- Choosing low-VOC or zero-VOC paints and environmentally friendly products whenever possible
- Seeking medical attention for evaluation and treatment of allergic reactions, especially in cases of severe or persistent symptoms

If someone suspects they have experienced an allergic reaction to paint, they should seek medical attention for proper evaluation and management. Allergy evaluation and management should be conducted under the guidance of a qualified healthcare professional, such as an allergist or dermatologist.

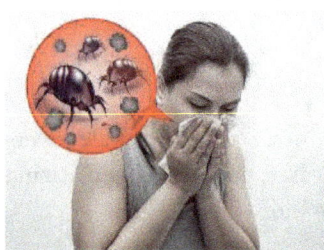

The Dust Allergy Index is a measure used to gauge the severity of dust allergens in the environment. Dust allergies are primarily caused by dust mites, microscopic organisms commonly found in household dust. Dust mites thrive in warm, humid environments and feed on organic matter like dead skin cells.

The Dust Allergy Index typically provides information about the concentration of dust mite allergens in the air, helping individuals with dust allergies anticipate and manage their symptoms. Here's a general overview of how the Dust Allergy Index works:

Measurement of Dust Allergen Levels: Dust allergen levels are measured using specialized equipment that collects air samples and detects the presence of dust mite particles or their waste products. Common methods for measuring dust allergens include enzyme-linked immunosorbent assay (ELISA) tests or immunoassay *techniques.*

- Classification of Dust Allergen Levels: Dust allergen levels are usually categorized into different levels based on the concentration of allergens detected in the air. These categories may include low, moderate, high, and very high levels of dust allergens.

- Forecasting: Dust Allergy Index may include forecasts that predict dust allergen levels for upcoming days or weeks. These forecasts take into account factors such as weather conditions, seasonal patterns, and historical data on dust allergen levels.

- Presentation of Information: Dust Allergy Index typically presents information about allergen levels in the form of charts, graphs, or maps that show trends over time or across different geographic regions. This information may be accessible through websites, mobile apps, or local health agencies.

- Guidance for Allergy Management: Dust Allergy Index often provides recommendations and tips for managing allergy symptoms during periods of high dust allergen levels. This may include advice on reducing exposure to dust allergens indoors, such as using allergen-proof bedding, vacuuming regularly, and using air purifiers with HEPA filters.

By staying informed about dust allergen levels and taking proactive steps to reduce exposure, individuals with dust allergies can better manage their symptoms and improve their quality of life, even during peak allergy seasons. If someone suspects they have a dust allergy or experiences symptoms such as sneezing, nasal congestion, itchy eyes, or asthma exacerbations, they should seek medical evaluation and treatment from a qualified healthcare professional, such as an allergist or immunologist.

Factors can influence the severity of **smoke-related allergies**, including the density of smoke particles in the air, the type of particles present (such as from wildfires or indoor sources like cigarettes), and individual sensitivities to smoke.

To gauge the impact of smoke on allergies, people often rely on air quality indexes provided by local environmental agencies. These indexes typically measure various pollutants, including particulate matter (PM2.5 and PM10), ozone, carbon monoxide, and sulfur dioxide. When there are significant wildfires or other sources of smoke, these indexes may reflect elevated levels of particulate matter, which can exacerbate respiratory issues and allergies.

Individuals with smoke allergies should monitor air quality reports and take necessary precautions during periods of poor air quality, such as staying indoors with windows and doors closed, using air purifiers equipped with HEPA filters, and avoiding strenuous outdoor activities. Additionally, consulting with a healthcare provider for personalized advice and treatment options is advisable for managing smoke allergies effectively.

However, allergic reactions to hair dye are not uncommon, and the severity of reactions can vary greatly depending on individual sensitivities and the specific ingredients in the dye.

Hair dye allergies can manifest as skin irritation, redness, itching, swelling, or even more severe reactions such as blistering and anaphylaxis in rare cases. The risk of allergy is higher with certain types of hair dyes, particularly those containing paraphenylenediamine (PPD) or related chemicals.

To minimize the risk of allergic reactions to hair dye, individuals can:

Perform a patch test: Apply a small amount of the dye to a small area of skin (usually behind the ear or on the inner elbow) at least 48 hours before full application to check for any adverse reactions.

Choose alternatives: Consider using hair dyes labeled as "hypoallergenic" or "PPD-free" if you have a known sensitivity to certain chemicals.

Seek professional advice: Consult a dermatologist or allergist if you have a history of allergic reactions to hair dye or other products, especially if you're unsure about specific ingredients.

Follow instructions carefully: Always follow the manufacturer's instructions for applying hair dye, including proper ventilation and recommended exposure times.

Consider alternatives: Explore alternative hair coloring options such as henna or vegetable-based dyes, which may be less likely to cause allergic reactions in some individuals.

If you experience any signs of an allergic reaction after using hair dye, such as itching, redness, swelling, or difficulty breathing, seek medical attention immediately. An allergist or dermatologist can provide guidance on managing allergic reactions and recommend suitable alternatives for hair coloring.

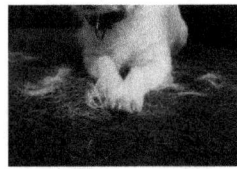

The presence of **animal fur** and dander can certainly trigger allergic reactions in susceptible individuals.

Allergic reactions to animal fur typically stem from proteins found in the animal's skin cells, urine, or saliva, rather than the fur itself. These proteins can become airborne and settle on surfaces throughout the home, leading to allergic symptoms when inhaled or upon contact with the skin.

Symptoms of animal fur allergies may include:

- Sneezing
- Runny or stuffy nose
- Itchy, watery eyes
- Skin rash or hives
- Asthma symptoms, such as coughing, wheezing, or chest tightness

To manage animal fur allergies effectively, individuals can take the following steps:

- Limit exposure: Minimize contact with animals known to trigger allergic reactions, such as cats, dogs, rabbits, or rodents. Consider keeping pets out of bedrooms and other areas where you spend a lot of time.

- Create allergen-free zones: Establish certain areas in the home where pets are not allowed, such as bedrooms or upholstered furniture, to reduce exposure to animal dander.

- Clean regularly: Vacuum carpets, rugs, and upholstery frequently using a vacuum cleaner equipped with a HEPA filter to trap allergens. Wash bedding, curtains, and other fabrics regularly in hot water to remove allergens.

- Use air purifiers: Consider using HEPA air purifiers in rooms where you spend a lot of time to help remove airborne allergens, including animal dander.

- Bathe pets regularly: Bathing pets regularly can help reduce the amount of dander they shed into the environment. Consult with a veterinarian for guidance on safe bathing practices for your pets.
- Consult an allergist: If you experience persistent or severe allergic symptoms despite taking preventive measures, consider consulting an allergist for allergy testing and personalized treatment options, such as allergy medications or immunotherapy.

While there isn't a specific index for animal fur allergies, individuals can monitor their symptoms and take proactive steps to minimize exposure to allergens in their environment.

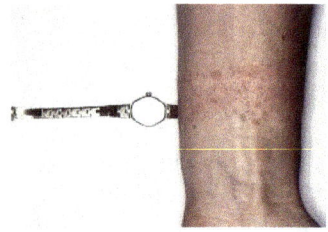

, particularly to certain metals commonly found in jewelry, are not uncommon.

Nickel, for example, is one of the most common allergens in metal jewelry. Allergic reactions to nickel can manifest as redness, itching, swelling, and even blistering or oozing at the site of contact. Other metals that may cause allergic reactions in sensitive individuals include cobalt, chromium, and copper.

To minimize the risk of allergic reactions to metal jewelry, individuals can take the following precautions:

- Choose hypoallergenic materials: Opt for jewelry made from hypoallergenic metals such as stainless steel, titanium, platinum, or gold (particularly 18 karat or higher, as lower karat gold may contain higher levels of allergenic metals like nickel).

- Avoid nickel-containing jewelry: If you have a known allergy to nickel, avoid wearing jewelry made from nickel or alloys containing nickel.

- Consider coatings or plating: Look for jewelry that is coated or plated with hypoallergenic materials like rhodium or palladium to create a barrier between the metal and your skin.

- Test jewelry before prolonged wear: Perform a patch test by wearing the jewelry on a small area of skin for a short period to check for any allergic reactions before wearing it for an extended period.

- Keep jewelry clean: Clean metal jewelry regularly with mild soap and water to remove any dirt, sweat, or other substances that may irritate the skin.

- Rotate jewelry: Avoid wearing the same piece of jewelry continuously, as prolonged exposure to metals may increase the risk of allergic reactions.

- Consult a dermatologist: If you experience persistent or severe allergic reactions to metal jewelry, consider consulting a dermatologist for allergy testing and personalized advice on managing metal allergies.

While there isn't an official index for metal jewelry allergies, individuals can take proactive measures to minimize the risk of allergic reactions by choosing jewelry made from hypoallergenic materials and avoiding metals known to cause allergies in sensitive individuals.

As of my last update in January 2022, there isn't a specific "seafood allergy index" comparable to pollen or air quality indexes. However, seafood allergies are a common type of food allergy and can cause a range of symptoms, from mild to severe, in affected individuals.

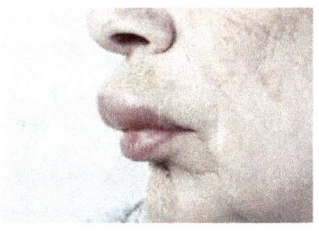

Seafood allergies can be triggered by various types of fish and shellfish, including but not limited to:

Fish: Examples include salmon, tuna, cod, and tilapia.

Shellfish: Examples include shrimp, crab, lobster, scallops, and clams.

Symptoms of a seafood allergy can include:

- Skin reactions such as hives, itching, or eczema
- Digestive symptoms like nausea, vomiting, or diarrhea
- Respiratory problems such as wheezing, coughing, or difficulty breathing
- Swelling of the lips, tongue, throat, or face (angioedema)

Anaphylaxis, a severe and potentially life-threatening allergic reaction characterized by a sudden drop in blood pressure, rapid pulse, and loss of consciousness

Managing a seafood allergy involves avoiding exposure to seafood and being vigilant about reading food labels and asking about ingredients in restaurant dishes. Cross-contact with seafood allergens can occur in shared cooking environments, so it's essential to communicate your allergy to food preparers.

In the absence of a specific seafood allergy index, individuals with seafood allergies should:

- Educate themselves about foods to avoid: Learn to recognize common seafood ingredients and dishes that may contain hidden seafood allergens.

- Carry emergency medication: Individuals with a history of severe allergic reactions should carry an epinephrine auto-injector (e.g., EpiPen) and know how to use it in case of anaphylaxis.

- Communicate with restaurant staff: Inform restaurant staff about your seafood allergy and ask about ingredients and cooking methods to ensure your meal is safe.

- Read food labels carefully: Check food labels for potential seafood allergens, even in unexpected products like sauces, soups, and condiments.

- Plan ahead when traveling: Research local cuisine and dining options at your destination to ensure you can find safe food choices.

If you suspect you have a seafood allergy or have experienced symptoms after consuming seafood, consult with a healthcare professional for diagnosis, management strategies, and personalized advice.

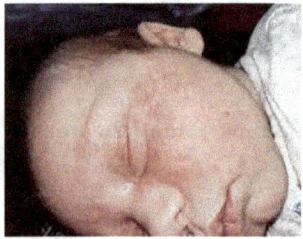

Milk allergies are one of the most common food allergies, particularly in children. An allergy to milk is an adverse immune response to one or more proteins found in cow's milk. It's important for individuals with a milk allergy to be aware of potential sources of milk proteins and to take precautions to avoid them.

Symptoms of a milk allergy can vary in severity and may include:

- Skin reactions such as hives, itching, or eczema
- Digestive symptoms like nausea, vomiting, diarrhea, or abdominal pain
- Respiratory problems such as wheezing, coughing, or difficulty breathing
- Swelling of the lips, tongue, throat, or face (angioedema)
- Anaphylaxis, a severe and potentially life-threatening allergic reaction characterized by a sudden drop in blood pressure, rapid pulse, and loss of consciousness

To manage a milk allergy effectively, individuals should:

- Read food labels carefully: Milk and milk products can be found in a wide range of foods and ingredients, including baked goods, processed meats, salad dressings, and snack foods. Check food labels for common milk-derived ingredients such as milk, lactose, casein, whey, and butter.

- Be cautious when dining out: Inform restaurant staff about your milk allergy and ask about ingredients and potential cross-contamination risks in menu items.

- Seek alternative sources of nutrients: Individuals with a milk allergy may need to find alternative sources of calcium, vitamin D, and other nutrients typically found in dairy products. Fortified plant-based milk alternatives and dietary supplements may be suitable options.

- Educate others: Make sure family members, caregivers, teachers, and others involved in your care are aware of your milk allergy and understand how to recognize and respond to allergic reactions.

- Carry emergency medication: Individuals with a history of severe allergic reactions should carry an epinephrine auto-injector (e.g., EpiPen) and know how to use it in case of anaphylaxis.

If you suspect you or someone you know has a milk allergy, consult with a healthcare professional for diagnosis, management strategies, and personalized advice. An allergist can perform tests to confirm a milk allergy and provide guidance on avoiding milk proteins and managing allergic reactions.

OBESITY

Abnormal lipid metabolism coefficient refers to a measure or coefficient related to abnormal lipid metabolism.

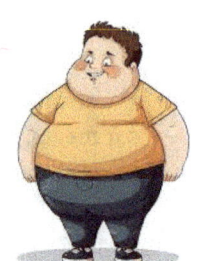

Lipid metabolism refers to the biochemical processes involved in the synthesis, breakdown, and transport of lipids (fats) in the body. Abnormal lipid metabolism can lead to various health issues, including dyslipidemia (abnormal levels of lipids in the blood), atherosclerosis (hardening and narrowing of the arteries), and cardiovascular disease.

When assessing lipid metabolism, healthcare providers typically measure various lipid parameters, including:

- Total cholesterol: The total amount of cholesterol in the blood, including both high-density lipoprotein (HDL) cholesterol and low-density lipoprotein (LDL) cholesterol.

- HDL cholesterol: Often referred to as "good" cholesterol because it helps remove LDL cholesterol from the bloodstream.

- LDL cholesterol: Often referred to as "bad" cholesterol because high levels are associated with an increased risk of atherosclerosis and cardiovascular disease.

- Triglycerides: A type of fat found in the blood that serves as an energy source for the body. Elevated triglyceride levels are also associated with an increased risk of cardiovascular disease.

There are various ratios and coefficients used to assess lipid metabolism and cardiovascular risk, such as the LDL/HDL ratio or the atherogenic index of plasma

(AIP). These measures provide insights into the balance between different lipid fractions and their impact on cardiovascular health.

Additionally, consulting with a healthcare professional or lipid specialist would be advisable for personalized assessment and management of lipid metabolism abnormalities.

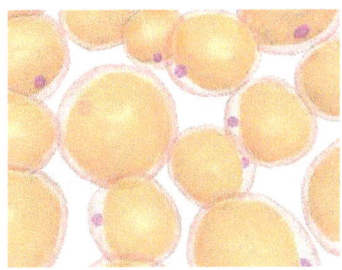

Brown adipose tissue refers to the fat tissue located in the brow region of the face.

While adipose tissue abnormalities can occur in various parts of the body and may be associated with conditions like obesity or lipodystrophy, specific abnormalities in brow adipose tissue may not be commonly studied or described using a coefficient.

If you're interested in understanding abnormalities in brow adipose tissue or any related conditions, I recommend consulting with a healthcare professional, particularly a dermatologist, plastic surgeon, or researcher specializing in facial anatomy or adipose tissue disorders. They can provide more information and guidance based on your specific concerns or interests.

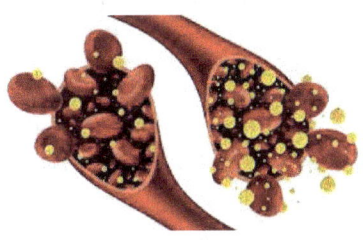

Hyperinsulinemia is a condition characterized by higher than normal levels of insulin in the blood. Insulin is a hormone produced by the pancreas that helps regulate blood sugar levels by facilitating the uptake of glucose into cells for energy or storage. Hyperinsulinemia can occur due to various factors, including insulin resistance (a condition in which cells become less responsive to insulin), obesity, certain medications, and certain medical conditions.

While there isn't a specific coefficient associated with hyperinsulinemia in mainstream medical terminology, healthcare providers may assess insulin levels through blood tests, such as fasting insulin levels or glucose tolerance tests. These tests help evaluate insulin resistance and assess the risk of conditions like type 2 diabetes and metabolic syndrome.

If you're concerned about hyperinsulinemia or related conditions, I recommend consulting with a healthcare professional, particularly an endocrinologist or a healthcare provider specializing in metabolic disorders. They can perform appropriate evaluations, interpret relevant tests, and provide personalized advice and treatment options based on your individual health status and needs.

The term "nucleus of the **hypothalamus abnormal coefficient**" appears to be a concatenation of several anatomical and medical concepts related to the hypothalamus, a crucial structure in the brain involved in various functions, including hormone regulation, temperature regulation, hunger, thirst, and circadian rhythms.

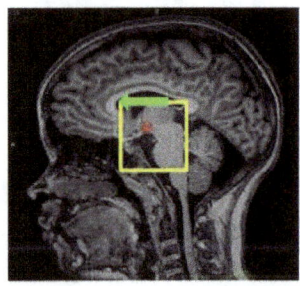

The hypothalamus contains several nuclei, each with specific functions and roles in regulating different physiological processes. Abnormalities within the hypothalamus or its nuclei can lead to various health issues, including disruptions in hormone regulation, appetite control, and sleep-wake cycles.

However, "abnormal coefficient" isn't a standard medical term in this context. Coefficients typically refer to numerical factors or values used in mathematical or statistical calculations, not anatomical structures or abnormalities.

Understanding the specific nature of any hypothalamic abnormalities and their potential implications typically requires a comprehensive evaluation, including medical history, physical examination, imaging studies (such as MRI or CT scans), and possibly laboratory tests.

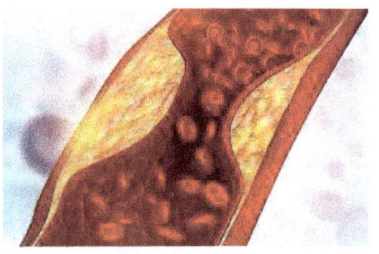

Triglycerides are a type of fat (lipid) found in your blood. They store excess energy from your diet and are an essential source of energy for your body. Abnormal levels of triglycerides can indicate an increased risk of heart disease and other health issues.

However, "triglyceride content of abnormal coefficient" is not a standard medical term or concept. It's possible you're referring to triglyceride levels being abnormal and being expressed as a coefficient or ratio in a particular context.

In medical practice, triglyceride levels are typically measured in milligrams per deciliter (mg/dL) or millimoles per liter (mmol/L) of blood. The normal range for triglycerides in adults is typically considered to be less than 150 mg/dL (or less than 1.7 mmol/L). Levels between 150 and 199 mg/dL (1.8 to 2.2 mmol/L) are considered borderline high, and levels of 200 mg/dL (2.3 mmol/L) or higher are considered high.

While there are various ratios and coefficients used in medicine to assess cardiovascular risk and lipid metabolism, such as the triglyceride to HDL cholesterol ratio, these are typically derived from triglyceride and cholesterol measurements and are not referred to as "triglyceride content of abnormal coefficient."

SKIN

Free radicals are unstable molecules that can damage cells and contribute to aging and various health issues, including skin aging and damage. In the context of skin health, free radicals can be generated by factors such as UV radiation, pollution, and smoking.

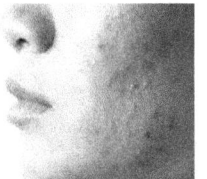

However, there are various methods and techniques used to assess oxidative stress and free radical damage in the skin. *These may include:*

- Biomarkers: Researchers may measure specific biomarkers of oxidative stress and free radical damage in the skin, such as levels of reactive oxygen species (ROS) or lipid peroxidation products.

- Imaging techniques: Advanced imaging techniques, such as electron paramagnetic resonance (EPR) spectroscopy or fluorescence microscopy, can be used to visualize and quantify free radicals and oxidative damage in skin tissues.

- Skin analysis devices: Some skincare devices claim to measure skin antioxidant levels or free radical activity using non-invasive methods such as spectrophotometry or impedance spectroscopy. However, the accuracy and reliability of these devices may vary, and their clinical significance may be limited.

- Clinical evaluation: Dermatologists may assess skin health and signs of oxidative stress during clinical examinations, such as evaluating skin texture, elasticity, pigmentation, and the presence of wrinkles or fine lines.

While there isn't a specific index or measurement widely recognized as a "skin free radical index," ongoing research aims to better understand the role of oxidative stress and free radicals in skin aging and disease. Protecting the skin from environmental factors that generate free radicals, such as UV radiation and pollution, and incorporating antioxidant-rich skincare products and a healthy lifestyle may help mitigate oxidative damage and support skin health.

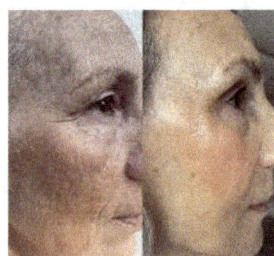

Collagen is a crucial protein found in the skin that provides structural support, elasticity, and strength. As we age, collagen production naturally decreases, leading to changes in skin texture, firmness, and appearance.

While there isn't a specific index called the "skin collagen index," various methods and techniques can assess collagen levels or collagen-related parameters in the skin:

- Biopsy and histology: Skin biopsies can be analyzed histologically to evaluate collagen content, organization, and quality. Techniques such as Masson's trichrome staining or picrosirius red staining can visualize collagen fibers and assess collagen density and distribution.

- Imaging techniques: Non-invasive imaging techniques, such as ultrasound, optical coherence tomography (OCT), or reflectance confocal microscopy (RCM), can be used to visualize and quantify collagen structure and density in the skin. These techniques provide insights into collagen organization and changes associated with aging, sun damage, or skin diseases.

- Biomarkers: Researchers may measure specific biomarkers related to collagen synthesis, degradation, or turnover in the skin. For example, levels of collagen-related proteins or enzymes (e.g., procollagen, matrix metalloproteinase) in skin samples or body fluids (e.g., blood, urine) can provide information about collagen metabolism and turnover.

- Clinical evaluation: Dermatologists and skincare professionals may assess skin collagen levels and quality during clinical examinations, such as evaluating skin firmness, elasticity, wrinkles, and sagging. While subjective, these evaluations can provide valuable insights into skin aging and collagen loss.

While there isn't a standardized "skin collagen index," these methods and techniques can provide valuable information about collagen levels, structure, and quality in the skin. Understanding collagen dynamics and the factors influencing collagen synthesis and degradation can inform skincare practices and interventions aimed at maintaining or enhancing skin health and appearance.

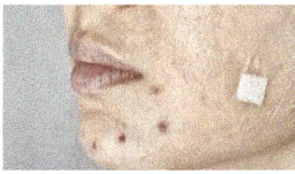

Skin grease index refer to the amount of sebum or oil present on the skin's surface. Sebum is an oily substance produced by the sebaceous glands in the skin and plays a role in keeping the skin lubricated and protected.

While there isn't a specific "skin grease index" measurement used in medical practice, skincare professionals may assess skin oiliness or sebum production using *various methods:*

- Visual assessment: Clinicians may visually inspect the skin to evaluate its appearance and oiliness. Oily skin often appears shiny or greasy, particularly in the T-zone (forehead, nose, and chin).
- Sebummetry: Sebummetry is a technique used to quantify sebum production by measuring the amount of oil present on the skin's surface. This can be done using specialized instruments such as a sebumeter, which uses absorbent materials or sensors to collect sebum from the skin's surface.

- Skin type classification: Skincare professionals often classify skin types based on oiliness, with categories such as dry, normal, combination, or oily skin. This classification helps guide skincare recommendations and product selection.

- Patient history: Clinicians may inquire about a patient's history of oily skin, acne, or other skin conditions to assess sebum production and skin health.

Excessively oily skin can contribute to issues such as acne, clogged pores, and shine, while too little sebum can lead to dryness and irritation. Proper skincare practices, such as gentle cleansing, moisturizing, and using products formulated for your skin type, can help maintain a healthy balance of sebum and promote skin health.

If you have concerns about oily skin or skin greasiness, consulting with a dermatologist or skincare professional can provide personalized recommendations and treatment options tailored to your needs.

The skin does play a crucial role in the body's immune system, serving as a barrier to protect against pathogens, toxins, and environmental insults.

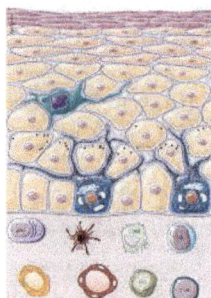

The skin's immune system is complex and involves various components, *including:*

- Physical barrier: The outermost layer of the skin, known as the stratum corneum, acts as a physical barrier that prevents the entry of harmful substances and microorganisms.
- Innate immunity: Skin cells such as keratinocytes, dendritic cells, and macrophages play important roles in innate immunity, which provides immediate, non-specific defense against pathogens.

- Adaptive immunity: The skin is also involved in adaptive immunity, which provides specific, targeted responses to pathogens encountered by the body.

Langerhans cells, a type of dendritic cell found in the skin, help initiate adaptive immune responses by presenting antigens to T cells.

- Immunomodulatory functions: The skin contains various molecules and cells involved in regulating immune responses and inflammation, such as cytokines, chemokine, and regulatory T cells.

While there isn't a specific "skin immunity index," researchers may study various aspects of skin immunity using techniques such as immunohistochemistry, flow cytometry, gene expression analysis, and cytokine profiling. These studies help understand how the skin's immune system responds to infections, allergens, autoimmune conditions, and other challenges.

Maintaining skin health and supporting the immune function of the skin involves practices such as proper hygiene, moisturizing, protecting the skin from UV radiation, and avoiding irritants and allergens. Additionally, consuming a balanced diet, getting enough sleep, managing stress, and avoiding smoking can help support overall immune function, including the skin's immune defenses.

If you have concerns about your skin's immune function or are experiencing skin-related issues, consulting with a dermatologist or immunologist can provide personalized evaluation and recommendations for maintaining skin health and immunity.

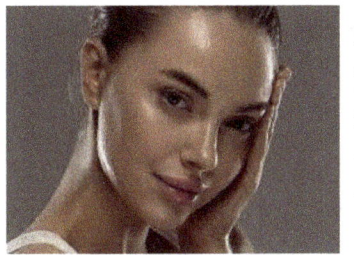

The "**skin moisture index**" refers to a measure of the hydration level or moisture content of the skin. Maintaining adequate skin hydration is essential for skin health and function, as it helps support the skin's barrier function, elasticity, and overall appearance.

There are various methods and devices used to assess skin moisture levels or hydration status:

- Corneometry: Corneometry is a common method used to measure skin hydration non-invasively. It involves using a corneometry, a device that measures the electrical capacitance of the skin, which correlates with the water content of the stratum corneum (the outermost layer of the skin).

- Conductance measurement: This method assesses skin hydration by measuring the skin's electrical conductivity, which is influenced by the water content of the skin.

- Moisture meters: Handheld moisture meters, often used in skincare clinics or beauty salons, use various techniques such as bio impedance or infrared spectroscopy to measure skin hydration levels.

- Visual assessment: Clinicians may visually inspect the skin to evaluate its appearance and hydration status. Dehydrated skin may appear dull, rough, or flaky, while well-hydrated skin typically looks smooth, plump, and radiant.

- Self-assessment scales: Patients may use self-assessment scales or questionnaires to subjectively evaluate their skin hydration levels and comfort.

Measuring skin moisture levels can help assess skin hydration, monitor changes over time, and guide skincare recommendations and treatments. Factors such as environmental conditions, skincare habits, diet, age, and underlying skin conditions can influence skin hydration levels.

To maintain optimal skin hydration and moisture balance, it's important to:

- Drink plenty of water: Staying hydrated from within by drinking an adequate amount of water throughout the day can help support overall skin health and hydration.

- Use moisturizers: Applying moisturizers regularly can help replenish and lock in moisture, especially after bathing or washing the skin.

- Avoid harsh skincare products: Limiting exposure to harsh soaps, cleansers, and skincare products that can strip the skin of its natural oils and disrupt the skin barrier.

- Protect the skin: Using sunscreen and protective clothing to shield the skin from UV radiation and environmental stressors can help prevent moisture loss and maintain skin hydration.

If you have concerns about your skin hydration levels or are experiencing dryness or dehydration, consulting with a dermatologist or skincare professional can provide personalized assessment and recommendations for improving skin moisture and hydration.

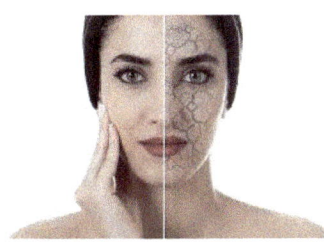

Skin moisture loss, also known as transepidermal water loss (TEWL), refers to the process by which water evaporates from the skin's surface into the surrounding environment. While some degree of moisture loss is normal and necessary for maintaining proper skin hydration, excessive or prolonged moisture loss can lead to dryness, dehydration, and impaired skin barrier function.

Several factors can contribute to skin moisture loss:

- Environmental factors: Low humidity levels, exposure to dry air, wind, and extreme temperatures can accelerate moisture evaporation from the skin, leading to increased TEWL.

- Harsh skincare products: Cleansers, soaps, and skincare products containing harsh detergents, alcohol, or fragrances can strip the skin of its natural oils and disrupt the skin barrier, contributing to moisture loss.

- Over washing: Frequent washing with hot water and harsh cleansers can remove the skin's natural oils and disrupt its protective barrier, leading to increased moisture loss.

- Aging: As we age, the skin's natural moisture barrier weakens, and the production of sebum (skin oil) decreases, making the skin more prone to moisture loss and dryness.

- Skin conditions: Certain skin conditions, such as eczema, psoriasis, and atopic dermatitis, can compromise the skin barrier and increase susceptibility to moisture loss.

- Lifestyle factors: Factors such as smoking, poor nutrition, stress, and inadequate hydration can affect skin health and contribute to moisture loss.

To help prevent or minimize skin moisture loss, consider the following tips:

- Use gentle cleansers: Opt for mild, fragrance-free cleansers that won't strip the skin of its natural oils.

- Moisturize regularly: Apply moisturizers containing hydrating ingredients such as hyaluronic acid, glycerin, ceramides, and natural oils to help replenish and lock in moisture.

- Use a humidifier: Using a humidifier in your home or workplace can help maintain optimal indoor humidity levels and prevent excessive moisture loss from the skin.

- Limit exposure to harsh environmental conditions: Protect your skin from harsh weather conditions by wearing protective clothing, using sunscreen, and avoiding prolonged exposure to extreme temperatures, wind, and dry air.

- Stay hydrated: Drink plenty of water throughout the day to support overall skin hydration from within.

- Avoid hot showers: Limit exposure to hot water, which can strip the skin of its natural oils and increase moisture loss.

- Consider skincare products: Look for skincare products formulated specifically for dry or sensitive skin, and avoid products containing ingredients that may exacerbate dryness or irritation.

If you're experiencing persistent or severe skin dryness or moisture loss, consult with a dermatologist or skincare professional for personalized evaluation and recommendations tailored to your skin type and concerns

The presence or measurement of small amounts of blood in the skin.

If someone is referring to "red blood traces" on the skin, they may be observing small amounts of blood that have leaked from tiny blood vessels near the skin's surface. This can occur for various reasons, such as minor cuts, scratches, or irritation from scratching or rubbing the skin.

In a medical context, the presence of blood on the skin may also be indicative of underlying conditions such as eczema, psoriasis, dermatitis, or other skin disorders characterized by inflammation or damage to the skin barrier.

If you're noticing persistent or concerning amounts of blood on the skin, it's essential to consult with a healthcare professional, such as a dermatologist, for proper evaluation and diagnosis. They can assess your skin, discuss any symptoms or concerns you may have, and recommend appropriate treatment or management strategies based on the underlying cause

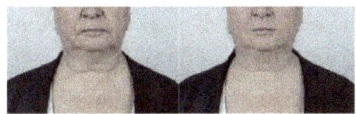

The "**skin elasticity index**" is a measurement used to assess the skin's ability to stretch and recoil, indicating its elasticity or resilience. Skin elasticity is an essential component of skin health and appearance, as it contributes to firmness, smoothness, and youthfulness.

Various methods and devices are used to measure skin elasticity:

- Cytometer: This device measures the skin's mechanical properties, including elasticity, firmness, and viscoelasticity. It applies suction to the skin and measures its deformation under controlled conditions.

- Extensometry: Extensometers are devices that measure the skin's ability to stretch and return to its original shape. They can be used to quantify parameters such as elasticity, tensile strength, and deformation.
- Ballistometer: Ballistometry is a technique that assesses skin elasticity by measuring the rebound of a small steel ball dropped onto the skin's surface.

- Imaging techniques: Advanced imaging techniques such as ultrasound elastography or optical coherence tomography (OCT) can visualize and quantify skin elasticity and mechanical properties.

- Clinical assessment: Dermatologists and skincare professionals may visually assess skin elasticity by gently pinching or pulling the skin and observing how quickly it returns to its original position.

Skin elasticity tends to decrease with age due to factors such as collagen and elastin degradation, decreased production of skin proteins, and changes in skin hydration. Sun exposure, smoking, poor nutrition, and other lifestyle factors can also affect skin elasticity.

Maintaining optimal skin elasticity involves practices such as protecting the skin from UV radiation, staying hydrated, eating a balanced diet rich in antioxidants and essential nutrients, avoiding smoking, and using skincare products containing ingredients that support collagen production and skin hydration.

If you're concerned about your skin's elasticity or noticing changes in skin firmness and resilience, consulting with a dermatologist or skincare professional can provide personalized evaluation and recommendations tailored to your skin type and concerns. They can recommend appropriate treatments, skincare products, and lifestyle modifications to help improve skin elasticity and maintain skin health.

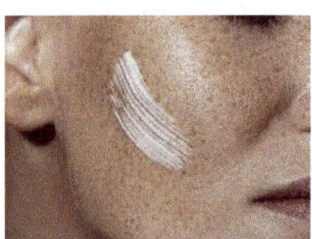

The "**skin melanin index**" refers to a measurement used to quantify the amount of melanin pigment present in the skin. Melanin is a pigment produced by melanocytes, specialized cells found in the skin, hair, and eyes. It plays a crucial role in determining skin color and provides protection against the harmful effects of ultraviolet (UV) radiation from the sun.

Several methods and devices can measure skin melanin levels or estimate skin pigmentation:

- Reflectance spectrophotometry: This technique measures the amount of light reflected or absorbed by the skin at specific wavelengths. Skin melanin levels can be estimated based on the degree of light absorption at different wavelengths.

- Colorimetry: Colorimeters are devices that measure color intensity and can be used to assess skin pigmentation. They may use standardized color scales or colorimetric indices to quantify melanin levels.

- Hexameter: The Hexameter is a handheld device that measures skin color and melanin levels by analyzing light absorption and reflection on the skin's surface.

- Skin biopsy: In research or clinical settings, skin biopsies can be performed to obtain tissue samples for histological analysis. Histological examination allows direct visualization of melanocytes and melanin pigmentation in the skin.

- Visual assessment: Clinicians may visually assess skin pigmentation using standardized scales or grading systems based on color intensity or distribution.

Skin melanin levels vary widely among individuals and are influenced by factors such as genetics, ethnicity, sun exposure, hormonal factors, and aging. Higher melanin levels provide greater protection against UV radiation and decrease the risk of sunburn and skin cancer. However, excessive sun exposure can lead to uneven pigmentation, sunspots, and other signs of sun damage.

Understanding skin melanin levels and pigmentation patterns is important for assessing skin health, diagnosing pigmentation disorders (such as hyperpigmentation or hypopigmentation), and guiding sun protection and skincare recommendations.

If you're concerned about your skin pigmentation or want to assess your skin's melanin levels, consulting with a dermatologist or skincare professional can provide personalized evaluation and recommendations based on your skin type, concerns, and medical history. They can recommend appropriate treatments, skincare products, and sun protection strategies to help maintain healthy and radiant skin.

It may refer to the degree of skin thickness or the presence of excess dead skin cells on the skin's surface, often described as "skin roughness" or "skin texture."

The outermost layer of the skin, known as the stratum corneum, is composed of dead skin cells (coenocytes) embedded in a lipid matrix. This layer acts as a barrier, protecting the underlying layers of the skin from environmental stressors and preventing moisture loss. The thickness and integrity of the stratum corneum are essential for maintaining skin health and function.

Several factors can contribute to changes in skin thickness or the accumulation of dead skin cells:

- Dryness: Inadequate hydration or exposure to harsh environmental conditions can lead to dry, rough skin and the accumulation of dead skin cells.
- Exfoliation: Insufficient exfoliation or ineffective removal of dead skin cells can result in a buildup of keratinized cells on the skin's surface, contributing to roughness and dullness.
- Aging: As we age, the turnover rate of skin cells decreases, resulting in a slower shedding of dead skin cells and potential thickening of the stratum corneum.
- Sun exposure: Chronic sun exposure can lead to thickening of the skin and the development of a rough, leathery texture, particularly in areas exposed to the sun.
- Skin conditions: Certain skin conditions, such as psoriasis, eczema, or keratosis pilaris, can cause rough, bumpy skin texture due to abnormal keratinization or inflammation.

To address rough skin texture and promote smoother, healthier skin, consider the following tips:

- Moisturize: Use moisturizers containing humectants and emollients to hydrate the skin and soften rough areas.

- Exfoliate: Incorporate gentle exfoliation into your skincare routine to remove dead skin cells and promote skin renewal. This can be done using physical exfoliates (such as scrubs or brushes) or chemical exfoliates (such as alpha hydroxyl acids or beta hydroxyl acids).

- Protect from the sun: Apply broad-spectrum sunscreen daily to protect the skin from UV damage and prevent thickening of the skin.

- Hydrate: Drink plenty of water to maintain skin hydration from within and support skin health.

- Seek professional advice: If you're concerned about rough skin texture or skin conditions affecting skin health, consult with a dermatologist or skincare professional for personalized evaluation and recommendations.

While there isn't a specific "skin horniness index," addressing factors that contribute to rough skin texture can help improve skin health and appearance.

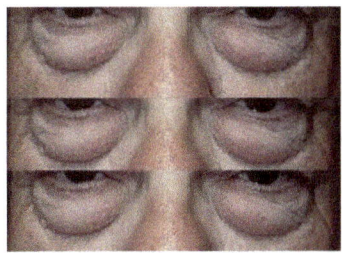

Bags under the eyes, also known as under-eye bags or periorbital puffiness, refer to swelling or puffiness in the area beneath the eyes. This condition can give the appearance of "bags" or bulges under the eyes, often creating a tired or aged appearance. *Under-eye bags can be caused by various factors, including:*

- Aging: As we age, the skin and tissues around the eyes may weaken, leading to a loss of elasticity and firmness. This can result in the accumulation of fat and fluid under the eyes, contributing to the appearance of under-eye bags.

- Genetics: Some individuals may be more prone to under-eye bags due to genetic factors. Genetics can influence the structure and thickness of the skin, as well as the distribution of fat and tissue around the eyes.

- Fluid retention: Fluid retention, often caused by factors like dietary habits, hormonal changes, allergies, or certain medical conditions, can lead to swelling and puffiness under the eyes.

- Allergies: Allergic reactions can cause inflammation and swelling in the delicate skin around the eyes, resulting in the appearance of under-eye bags.

- Fatigue and lack of sleep: Insufficient sleep or poor sleep quality can contribute to fluid retention and swelling under the eyes, exacerbating the appearance of under-eye bags.

- Lifestyle factors: Factors such as smoking, excessive alcohol consumption, sun exposure, and poor skincare habits can contribute to skin aging and the development of under-eye bags.

While under-eye bags are often a cosmetic concern rather than a medical issue, they can affect one's appearance and self-confidence. Treatment options for under-eye bags may include:

- Lifestyle changes: Getting an adequate amount of sleep, managing stress, staying hydrated, maintaining a healthy diet, and avoiding smoking and excessive alcohol consumption can help reduce the appearance of under-eye bags.

- Topical treatments: Over-the-counter or prescription skincare products containing ingredients such as retinol, vitamin C, caffeine, hyaluronic acid, and peptides may help improve the appearance of under-eye bags by promoting collagen production, increasing skin firmness, and reducing inflammation.

- Cosmetic procedures: In some cases, cosmetic procedures such as injectable fillers, laser therapy, chemical peels, or surgical procedures like blepharoplasty (eyelid surgery) may be recommended to address more severe or persistent under-eye bags.

If you're concerned about under-eye bags or other cosmetic issues affecting the appearance of your eyes, consulting with a dermatologist or cosmetic surgeon can provide personalized evaluation and recommendations for treatment options tailored to your needs and goals.

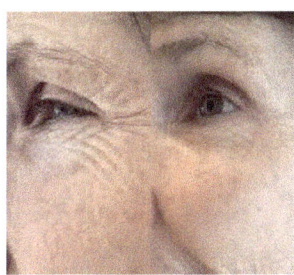

Collagen plays a crucial role in maintaining the skin's structure, firmness, and elasticity. As we age, the production of collagen decreases, leading to the formation of wrinkles and fine lines, including those around the eyes. Eye wrinkles, also known as crow's feet or periorbital wrinkles, are lines that develop at the outer corners of the eyes and are often associated with aging and repeated facial expressions.

Several factors contribute to the formation of collagen eye wrinkles:

- Aging: The natural aging process leads to a decrease in collagen production and skin elasticity, making the skin more prone to wrinkles and fine lines.

- Sun exposure: Ultraviolet (UV) radiation from the sun accelerates collagen breakdown and damages the skin's structure, contributing to the formation of wrinkles, including those around the eyes.

- Facial expressions: Repeated facial expressions, such as squinting or smiling, can cause creases and lines to form in the skin over time, leading to the development of eye wrinkles.

- Lifestyle factors: Factors such as smoking, poor nutrition, inadequate hydration, and chronic stress can also affect collagen production and skin health, making the skin more susceptible to wrinkles.

While it's not possible to completely eliminate eye wrinkles, there are several strategies to help reduce their appearance and prevent further damage:

- Use sunscreen: Apply a broad-spectrum sunscreen with a minimum SPF of 30 to protect the delicate skin around the eyes from UV damage and prevent collagen breakdown.

- Moisturize: Use a hydrating eye cream or moisturizer containing ingredients such as hyaluronic acid, peptides, and antioxidants to keep the skin around the eyes moisturized and plump.

- Avoid smoking: Smoking accelerates skin aging and collagen breakdown, leading to the formation of wrinkles. Quitting smoking can help improve skin health and reduce the appearance of eye wrinkles.

- Wear sunglasses: Wear sunglasses with UV protection to shield the eyes from harmful UV radiation and minimize squinting, which can contribute to the development of eye wrinkles.

- Use retinoids: Topical retinoids, such as retinol or prescription retinoids like retinoid, can help stimulate collagen production and improve the appearance of fine lines and wrinkles around the eyes over time.

- Consider cosmetic procedures: Cosmetic procedures such as injectable fillers, botulinum toxin (Botox) injections, laser therapy, or chemical peels may be options for reducing the appearance of eye wrinkles, depending on individual preferences and goals.

It's important to note that consistency and patience are key when addressing eye wrinkles, as results may take time to become noticeable. If you have concerns about eye wrinkles or are considering treatment options, consulting with a dermatologist or skincare professional can provide personalized evaluation and recommendations tailored to your needs and goals.

Dark circles under the eyes, also known as periorbital dark circles, are a common cosmetic concern that can affect people of all ages and skin types. They appear as dark or discolored areas beneath the eyes and are often accompanied by

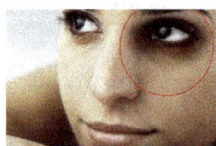

puffiness or hollowing in the under-eye area. *Several factors can contribute to the development of dark circles:*

- Genetics: Genetics plays a significant role in the development of dark circles. Some individuals inherit thinner skin or increased pigmentation around the eyes, making blood vessels and underlying structures more visible, resulting in a darker appearance.

- Thin skin: The skin around the eyes is thinner and more delicate than skin in other areas of the body. Thinner skin allows blood vessels and underlying structures, such as fat pads and muscles, to be more visible, leading to the appearance of dark circles.

- Fatigue and lack of sleep: Inadequate sleep or poor sleep quality can cause blood vessels to dilate and become more visible beneath the thin skin around the eyes, resulting in dark circles. Additionally, fatigue can lead to paleness or a sallow complexion, making dark circles more noticeable.

- Aging: As we age, the skin around the eyes becomes thinner and loses collagen and elasticity, making blood vessels and pigmentation more visible. Loss of fat and volume in the *under-eye area can also contribute to hollowing and the appearance of dark circles.*

- Sun exposure: Chronic sun exposure can lead to hyperpigmentation and the overproduction of melanin in the skin, resulting in darkening of the under-eye area.

- Allergies: Allergic reactions, such as hay fever or allergic rhinitis, can cause inflammation and swelling around the eyes, leading to dark circles. Rubbing or scratching the eyes due to allergies can also worsen the appearance of dark circles.

- Lifestyle factors: Factors such as smoking, excessive alcohol consumption, dehydration, and poor nutrition can contribute to the development of dark circles by affecting skin health and circulation.

While dark circles are often a cosmetic concern rather than a medical issue, *several strategies can help reduce their appearance*:

- Get enough sleep: Aim for 7-9 hours of quality sleep each night to minimize fatigue and improve overall skin health.

- Manage allergies: Take steps to minimize exposure to allergens and seek treatment for allergy symptoms to reduce inflammation and swelling around the eyes.

- Protect your skin: Apply sunscreen daily and wear sunglasses to protect the delicate skin around the eyes from UV damage and pigmentation.

- Use topical treatments: Use skincare products containing ingredients such as vitamin C, retinoid, kojic acid, niacinamide, and caffeine to brighten and tighten the under-eye area, reduce pigmentation, and improve skin texture.

- Use cold compresses: Apply cold compresses or chilled cucumber slices to the eyes to constrict blood vessels, reduce inflammation, and temporarily improve the appearance of dark circles.

- Consider cosmetic procedures: Cosmetic procedures such as dermal fillers, laser therapy, chemical peels, or micro needling may be options for reducing the appearance of dark circles, depending on individual preferences and goals.

If you have persistent or severe dark circles that do not improve with lifestyle changes or over-the-counter treatments, consider consulting with a dermatologist or skincare professional for personalized evaluation and recommendations. They can help identify the underlying causes of dark circles and recommend appropriate treatment options tailored to your needs and goals.

Lymphatic obstruction around the eyes can lead to a condition known as periorbital lymphedema, which is characterized by swelling or puffiness in the tissues surrounding the eyes. The lymphatic system plays a crucial role in maintaining fluid balance and immune function by transporting lymphatic fluid, which contains white blood cells and waste products, throughout the body.

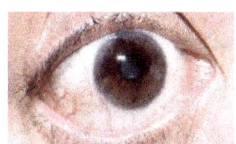

When the lymphatic vessels in the periorbital area become blocked or impaired, lymphatic fluid may accumulate, leading to swelling and puffiness around the eyes. Lymphatic obstruction around the eyes can occur due to various reasons, *including:*

- Surgery: Surgical procedures involving the eyes, face, or head, such as eyelid surgery, facial cosmetic surgery, or procedures to remove tumors, may disrupt the normal lymphatic drainage pathways and lead to lymphedema around the eyes.

- Trauma: Traumatic injuries, such as fractures or blunt force trauma to the face or head, can damage the lymphatic vessels and impair lymphatic drainage, resulting in periorbital lymphedema.

- Infection: Inflammatory conditions or infections affecting the eyes or surrounding tissues, such as cellulitis or orbital inflammation, can lead to swelling and lymphatic obstruction in the periorbital area.

- Radiation therapy: Radiation therapy for conditions such as cancer may damage the lymphatic vessels and impair lymphatic drainage, leading to lymphedema around the eyes as a side effect of treatment.

- Congenital abnormalities: Rare congenital conditions affecting the development or function of the lymphatic system, such as lymphatic malformations or primary lymphedema, can predispose individuals to lymphatic obstruction and swelling around the eyes.

Periorbital lymphedema can cause discomfort, tightness, and cosmetic concerns, and may also affect vision if severe swelling puts pressure on the eye structures. Treatment for lymphatic obstruction around the eyes may include:

- Manual lymphatic drainage: Gentle massage techniques performed by a trained therapist can help stimulate lymphatic flow and reduce swelling in the periorbital area.

- Compression therapy: Wearing compression garments or bandages around the eyes can help support lymphatic drainage and reduce swelling.

- Topical treatments: Topical medications containing ingredients such as hyaluronic acid, caffeine, or aminophylline may help improve lymphatic circulation and reduce fluid retention in the periorbital area.

- Surgical intervention: In severe cases of periorbital lymphedema that do not respond to conservative treatments, surgical procedures such as lymphatic venous anastomosis or lymph node transfer may be considered to restore lymphatic drainage and reduce swelling.

If you're experiencing persistent swelling or puffiness around the eyes, it's essential to consult with a healthcare professional, such as an ophthalmologist or dermatologist, for proper evaluation and diagnosis. They can help determine the underlying cause of the swelling and recommend appropriate treatment options tailored to your specific needs and circumstances.

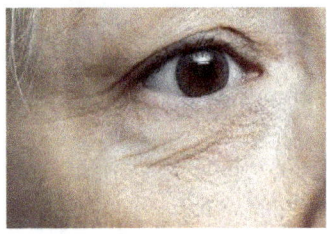

Sagging around the eyes, often referred to as "eyelid ptosis" or "drooping eyelids," is a common cosmetic concern that can affect both the upper and lower eyelids. It is characterized by a downward displacement or hooding of the eyelid skin, which can obscure the natural contours of the eyes and contribute to a tired or aged appearance. *Several factors can contribute to sagging around the eyes*:

- Aging: As we age, the skin and tissues around the eyes lose elasticity and firmness, leading to sagging and drooping of the eyelids. Additionally, weakening of the muscles that support the eyelids can exacerbate the problem.

- Genetics: Genetic factors can influence the rate at which the skin ages and the degree of sagging experienced around the eyes. Some individuals may be predisposed to develop sagging eyelids earlier or more prominently than others.

- Sun exposure: Chronic exposure to ultraviolet (UV) radiation from the sun accelerates skin aging and collagen breakdown, leading to loss of skin elasticity and firmness around the eyes.

- Lifestyle factors: Unhealthy lifestyle habits, such as smoking, poor nutrition, excessive alcohol consumption, and lack of sleep, can contribute to premature skin aging and exacerbate sagging around the eyes.

- Eyestrain and fatigue: Prolonged periods of eyestrain or fatigue, such as staring at digital screens for extended periods or not getting enough sleep, can weaken the muscles around the eyes and contribute to sagging eyelids.

Sagging around the eyes can be addressed through various treatment options, depending on the severity of the condition and individual preferences:

- Topical treatments: Skincare products containing ingredients such as retinoid, peptides, antioxidants, and moisturizers can help improve skin elasticity, texture, and firmness around the eyes.

- Botox injections: Botulinum toxin (Botox) injections can be used to temporarily relax the muscles around the eyes, reducing the appearance of dynamic wrinkles and lifting drooping eyelids.

- Dermal fillers: Injectable fillers containing hyaluronic acid or other biocompatible materials can be used to restore volume and support to the under-eye area, reducing the appearance of sagging and hollowing.

- Eyelid surgery (blepharoplasty): Surgical procedures such as upper or lower blepharoplasty can be performed to remove excess skin and fat, tighten the underlying muscles, and improve the overall contour and appearance of the eyelids.

- Radiofrequency or laser therapy: Non-invasive procedures such as radiofrequency or laser therapy can stimulate collagen production, tighten the skin, and improve sagging around the eyes.

If you're concerned about sagging around your eyes or considering treatment options, it's essential to consult with a board-certified dermatologist or oculoplastic surgeon. They can provide a comprehensive evaluation, discuss your goals and concerns, and recommend the most appropriate treatment options for achieving your desired results.

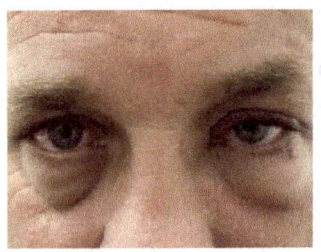

Edema is the medical term for swelling caused by excess fluid trapped in body tissues. When it occurs around the eyes, it's often referred to as periorbital edema or eyelid edema.

Periorbital edema can result from various factors:

- Allergies: Allergic reactions to pollen, dust, pet dander, or certain foods can cause inflammation and fluid retention around the eyes, leading to swelling.

- Sinusitis: Sinus infections or inflammation can cause congestion and fluid buildup in the sinus cavities, leading to periorbital edema.

- Lack of sleep: Insufficient sleep or poor sleep quality can lead to fluid retention and puffiness around the eyes.

- Dehydration: Inadequate hydration can cause the body to retain sodium, leading to water retention and periorbital edema.

- Eye strain: Prolonged periods of reading, staring at screens, or other activities that strain the eyes can contribute to fluid accumulation and swelling around the eyes.

- Injuries: Trauma or injuries to the eye area, such as blunt force trauma or surgery, can cause localized swelling and edema.

- Medical conditions: Certain medical conditions, such as thyroid disorders, kidney disease, heart failure, or liver disease, can cause fluid retention and edema throughout the body, including the periorbital area.

To reduce periorbital edema and alleviate swelling around the eyes, consider the following tips:

- Apply cold compresses: Applying cold compresses or chilled cucumber slices to the eyes can help constrict blood vessels and reduce swelling.

- Get enough sleep: Aim for 7-9 hours of quality sleep each night to minimize fluid retention and puffiness around the eyes.

- Stay hydrated: Drink plenty of water throughout the day to maintain proper hydration and prevent fluid retention.

- Elevate your head while sleeping: Sleeping with your head elevated can help reduce fluid accumulation in the periorbital area.

- Limit salt intake: Excess sodium in the diet can contribute to fluid retention, so try to minimize your intake of salty foods.

- Manage allergies: Take steps to minimize exposure to allergens and seek treatment for allergy symptoms to reduce inflammation and swelling around the eyes.

Use over-the-counter treatments: Over-the-counter antihistamines or decongestants may help alleviate allergy-related periorbital edema, but consult with a healthcare professional before using any medication.

If you're experiencing persistent or severe periorbital edema, or if it's accompanied by other concerning symptoms, it's essential to consult with a healthcare professional for proper evaluation and treatment. They can help determine the underlying cause of the edema and recommend appropriate management strategies based on your specific needs and medical history.

"**Eye cell activity**" could refer to the metabolic processes and functions of cells within the eyes. The eyes are complex organs composed of various types of cells, each with specific functions contributing to vision and overall eye health. *Here's an overview of some key cell types in the eyes and their activities:*

• Photoreceptor cells: Photoreceptor cells, including rods and cones, are located in the retina, the light-sensitive tissue lining the back of the eye. These cells detect light and convert it into electrical signals that are transmitted to the brain, where they are interpreted as visual images.

• Retinal ganglion cells: Retinal ganglion cells receive signals from photoreceptor cells and transmit them to the brain via the optic nerve. These cells play a crucial role in transmitting visual information and are involved in various visual functions, including contrast sensitivity, motion detection, and depth perception.

• Retinal pigment epithelial cells (RPE): RPE cells are located beneath the photoreceptor cells in the retina and perform several essential functions, including phagocytosis of photoreceptor outer segments, recycling of visual pigments, maintenance of the blood-retina barrier, and regulation of ion and fluid transport.

• Corneal epithelial cells: The cornea, the transparent outer covering of the eye, is composed of several layers of epithelial cells. Corneal epithelial cells play a crucial role in maintaining the integrity and clarity of the cornea, protecting the eye from injury and infection, and facilitating the passage of light into the eye.

- Lens epithelial cells: Lens epithelial cells are located in the lens, a transparent structure behind the iris that focuses light onto the retina. These cells play a role in lens growth and maintenance, as well as the production and maintenance of lens proteins called crystalline.

- Endothelial cells: Endothelial cells line the inner surface of blood vessels, including those in the eyes. In the cornea, endothelial cells help maintain corneal transparency by regulating fluid balance and removing excess fluid from the corneal stroma.

- Immune cells: Various immune cells, including macrophages, lymphocytes, and dendritic cells, are present in the eyes and play a role in immune surveillance, inflammation, and defense against pathogens.

The activity of these cells is tightly regulated and coordinated to maintain normal eye function and health. Disruptions or abnormalities in cellular activity can lead to various eye conditions and diseases, including age-related macular degeneration, diabetic retinopathy, glaucoma, cataracts, and corneal diseases. Understanding the cellular mechanisms underlying these conditions is essential for developing effective treatments and interventions to preserve vision and improve eye health.

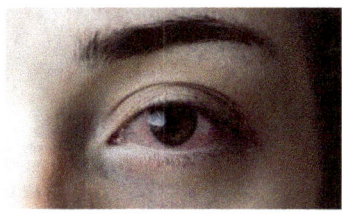

Visual fatigue, also known as eye strain or asthenopia, refers to discomfort or tiredness of the eyes that occurs after extended periods of focusing on a task, such as reading, using digital devices, or driving. It is a common condition that can affect people of all ages, particularly those who spend a significant amount of time performing near work activities.

Several factors can contribute to visual fatigue:

- Prolonged near work: Extended periods of reading, writing, or using digital devices can lead to focusing fatigue, as the eye muscles work harder to maintain clear vision at close distances.

- Poor lighting: Inadequate lighting conditions, such as dim lighting or glare from overhead lights or screens, can strain the eyes and contribute to visual fatigue.

- Improper ergonomics: Poor posture or improper positioning of screens or reading materials can lead to neck, shoulder, and eye strain, exacerbating visual fatigue.

- Uncorrected refractive errors: Refractive errors such as nearsightedness, farsightedness, or astigmatism can cause blurred vision and eye strain, particularly during near work tasks.

- Dry eyes: Insufficient tear production or excessive evaporation of tears can lead to dry eyes, causing discomfort, irritation, and visual fatigue.

- Digital eye strain: Excessive use of digital devices, such as smartphones, tablets, and computers, can lead to digital eye strain, characterized by symptoms such as eye discomfort, dryness, blurred vision, and headaches.

- Blue light exposure: Prolonged exposure to blue light emitted by digital screens, LED lights, and sunlight can disrupt the body's circadian rhythm, suppress melatonin production, and contribute to visual fatigue and sleep disturbances.

To reduce visual fatigue and prevent eye strain, consider the following tips:

- Take regular breaks: Follow the 20-20-20 rule - take a 20-second break every 20 minutes and look at something 20 feet away to relax and rest your eyes.

- Blink frequently: Blinking helps moisten the eyes and prevent dryness, so make a conscious effort to blink more often, especially when using digital devices.

- Adjust lighting: Ensure adequate lighting when reading or working, and minimize glare from screens or reflective surfaces by using anti-glare screens or adjusting screen brightness.
- Maintain proper ergonomics: Position screens or reading materials at a comfortable distance (about arm's length) and angle to reduce strain on the eyes and neck.

- Use proper eyewear: If you have refractive errors, wear corrective lenses as prescribed by your eye care professional to maintain clear vision and reduce eye strain.

- Stay hydrated: Drink plenty of water to maintain adequate tear production and prevent dry eyes.

- Limit screen time: Take regular breaks from digital devices and limit screen time, especially before bedtime, to reduce blue light exposure and promote better sleep.

If you experience persistent or severe visual fatigue despite these measures, or if you have other concerning symptoms such as eye pain, double vision, or vision changes, it's essential to consult with an eye care professional for proper evaluation and management. They can assess your eye health, identify any underlying issues contributing to visual fatigue, and recommend appropriate treatments or interventions to alleviate symptoms and promote eye comfort.

COLLAGEN

Eye illnesses encompass a wide range of conditions affecting the eyes, ranging from common and temporary issues to more severe and chronic diseases. Some of the *most common eye illnesses include:*

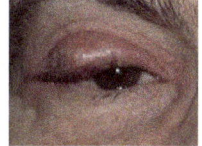

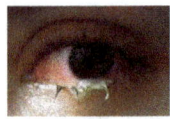
- Conjunctivitis (Pink Eye): Inflammation of the conjunctiva, the thin, transparent membrane covering the white part of the eye and inner eyelids. It can be caused by viruses, bacteria, allergens, or irritants.

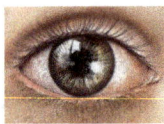
- Dry Eye Syndrome: A condition characterized by insufficient tear production or poor tear quality, leading to dryness, irritation, and discomfort in the eyes.

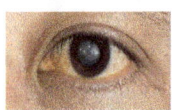
- Cataracts: Clouding of the lens of the eye, which leads to blurry vision, glare sensitivity, and difficulty seeing in low light conditions. Cataracts commonly occur with aging but can also result from trauma, medications, or underlying medical conditions.

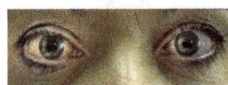
- Glaucoma: A group of eye diseases characterized by damage to the optic nerve, often caused by elevated intraocular pressure (fluid pressure inside the eye). Glaucoma can lead to vision loss and blindness if left untreated.

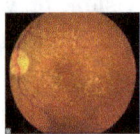
- Age-related Macular Degeneration (AMD): A progressive deterioration of the macula, the central part of the retina responsible for central vision. AMD is a leading cause of vision loss in older adults.

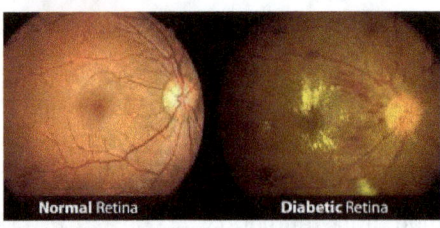
- Diabetic Retinopathy: A complication of diabetes that affects the blood vessels in the retina, leading to vision loss if left untreated. Diabetic retinopathy can cause hemorrhages, swelling, and abnormal blood vessel growth in the retina.

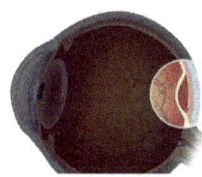
- Retinal Detachment: Separation of the retina from the underlying tissue, often caused by trauma, aging, or underlying eye conditions. Retinal detachment can cause sudden vision loss and requires prompt medical attention.

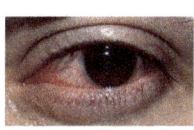
- Keratitis: Inflammation of the cornea, the transparent outer covering of the eye. Keratitis can be caused by infections, injuries, contact lens wear, or underlying medical conditions.

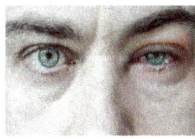
- Blepharitis: Inflammation of the eyelids, often associated with redness, swelling, itching, and crusting around the eyelashes. Blepharitis can result from bacterial or fungal infections, allergies, or underlying skin conditions.

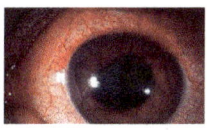
- Uveitis: Inflammation of the uvea, the middle layer of the eye that includes the iris, ciliary body, and choroid. Uveitis can cause eye pain, redness, light sensitivity, and vision changes.

These are just a few examples of eye illnesses, and there are many other conditions that can affect the eyes. If you're experiencing symptoms such as eye pain, redness, blurred vision, or changes in vision, it's essential to consult with an eye care professional for proper evaluation and treatment. Early detection and management of eye illnesses are crucial for preserving vision and preventing complications.

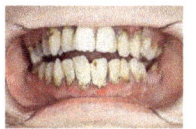
Tooth illnesses encompass a range of conditions affecting the teeth and surrounding structures in the mouth. Some common tooth illnesses *include:*

Tooth Decay (Cavities): Tooth decay is caused by bacteria in the mouth that produce acids that gradually erode the enamel, leading

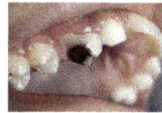

to the formation of cavities or holes in the teeth. If left untreated, tooth decay can progress and affect deeper layers of the tooth, leading to pain, infection, and tooth loss.

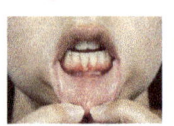
- Gum Disease (Periodontal Disease): Gum disease is an infection of the tissues surrounding and supporting the teeth, including the gums, periodontal ligaments, and alveolar bone. It typically starts with gingivitis, characterized by red, swollen gums that bleed easily, and can progress to periodontitis, which causes gum recession, bone loss, and tooth loosening.

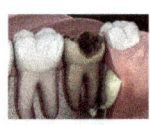
- Tooth Abscess: A tooth abscess is a pocket of pus that forms within the tooth or in the surrounding tissues due to a bacterial infection. It can cause severe pain, swelling, fever, and general discomfort.

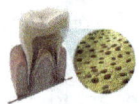
- Tooth Sensitivity: Tooth sensitivity occurs when the protective enamel layer of the tooth becomes worn down, exposing the underlying dentin and nerve endings. It can cause pain or discomfort when consuming hot, cold, sweet, or acidic foods and beverages.

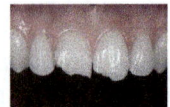
- Tooth Fractures: Tooth fractures can occur due to trauma, biting on hard objects, or weakening of the tooth structure from decay or large fillings. Depending on the severity of the fracture, it may cause pain, sensitivity, or compromise the structural integrity of the tooth.

- Tooth Erosion: Tooth erosion is the gradual loss of tooth enamel due to acid
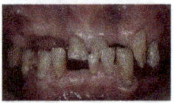
exposure from acidic foods and beverages, acid reflux, or excessive brushing. It can lead to tooth sensitivity, changes in tooth color, and increased risk of cavities.

- Tooth Grinding (Bruxism): Bruxism is the habit of clenching or grinding the teeth, often during sleep. It can lead to tooth wear, cracks, fractures, and jaw pain.

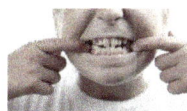
- Malocclusion: Malocclusion refers to misalignment of the teeth or improper positioning of the upper and lower jaws. It can cause difficulty chewing, speech problems and increased risk of tooth decay and gum disease.

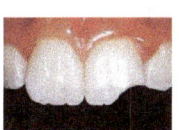
- Dental Trauma: Dental trauma can result from accidents, falls, or sports injuries, leading to fractures, displacement, or avulsion (complete loss) of teeth.

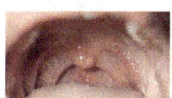
- Oral Cancer: Oral cancer can affect the lips, tongue, cheeks, and floor of the mouth, palate, and throat. Early signs may include persistent mouth sores, lumps, or patches, difficulty swallowing or chewing, and changes in voice.

These are just a few examples of tooth illnesses, and there are many other conditions that can affect dental health. Proper oral hygiene, regular dental check-ups, and prompt treatment of dental issues are essential for maintaining oral health and preventing complications. If you're experiencing any symptoms or concerns related to your dental health, it's important to consult with a dentist or oral healthcare professional for evaluation and appropriate management.

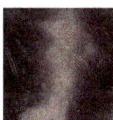
Hair and skin illnesses encompass a wide range of conditions affecting the hair follicles, scalp, skin, and associated structures. Some common hair and skin *illnesses include*:

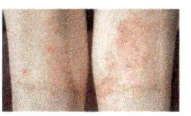
- Dermatitis: Dermatitis refers to inflammation of the skin, which can manifest as redness, itching, swelling, and scaling. Types of dermatitis include contact dermatitis (caused by contact with irritants or allergens), seborrheic dermatitis (affects areas rich in sebaceous glands, such as the scalp), and atopic dermatitis (eczema).

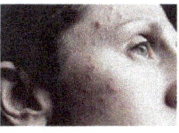
- Acne: Acne is a common skin condition characterized by the formation of pimples, blackheads, whiteheads, and cysts due to clogged pores, inflammation, and bacterial overgrowth. It often occurs on the face, chest, back, and shoulders.

- Psoriasis: Psoriasis is a chronic autoimmune condition that causes the rapid growth of skin cells, leading to the formation of thick, red, scaly patches on the skin. It commonly affects the scalp, elbows, knees, and lower back.

- Alopecia: Alopecia refers to hair loss or thinning that can occur on the scalp or other parts of the body. Types of alopecia include androgenetic alopecia (male-pattern or female-pattern baldness), alopecia areata (patches of hair loss), and telogen effluvium (excessive shedding due to stress, illness, or hormonal changes).

- Dandruff: Dandruff is a common scalp condition characterized by flaking and itching of the scalp. It can be caused by factors such as dry skin, fungal overgrowth (malassezia), or seborrheic dermatitis.

- Hives (Urticarial): Hives are raised, itchy welts that appear on the skin due to allergic reactions or other triggers, such as medications, insect bites, or stress.

- Eczema (Atopic Dermatitis): Eczema is a chronic inflammatory skin condition characterized by dry, itchy, red, and inflamed patches of skin. It often occurs in individuals with a personal or family history of allergies, asthma, or eczema.

- Tinea Infections: Tinea infections, also known as ringworm, are fungal infections of the skin, scalp, or nails. Common types include tinea corporis (ringworm of the body), tinea capitis (ringworm of the scalp), and tinea pedis (athlete's foot).

- Rosacea: Rosacea is a chronic skin condition that causes redness, flushing, visible blood vessels, and acne-like bumps on the face, particularly the cheeks, nose, chin, and forehead.

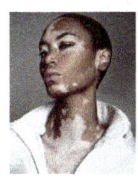
- Vitiligo: Vitiligo is a skin disorder characterized by the loss of skin pigment, resulting in white patches or depigmentation on the skin.

These are just a few examples of hair and skin illnesses, and there are many other conditions that can affect the hair and skin. Proper skincare, hair care, lifestyle modifications, and medical treatments are often necessary to manage these conditions effectively. If you're experiencing any symptoms or concerns related to your hair or skin health, it's important to consult with a dermatologist or healthcare professional for evaluation, diagnosis, and appropriate management.

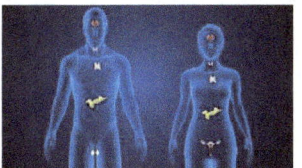
The endocrine system is a complex network of glands and organs that produce and release hormones, chemical messengers that regulate various physiological processes and maintain homeostasis within the body. Hormones travel through the bloodstream to target cells or organs, where they exert their effects by binding to specific receptors and initiating cellular responses.

Key components of the endocrine system include:

- Glands: Endocrine glands are specialized organs that produce and release hormones directly into the bloodstream. Major endocrine glands include the pituitary gland, thyroid gland, parathyroid glands, adrenal glands, pancreas, ovaries (in females), and testes (in males).

- Hormones: Hormones are signaling molecules produced by endocrine glands that regulate a wide range of physiological functions, including metabolism, growth and development, reproduction, stress response, immune function, and electrolyte balance.

- Hypothalamus: The hypothalamus is a small region of the brain located below the thalamus. It plays a crucial role in regulating hormone production by releasing signaling molecules called releasing hormones or inhibiting hormones, which stimulate or inhibit the secretion of hormones from the pituitary gland.

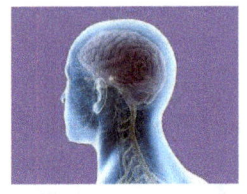

- Pituitary Gland: Often referred to as the "master gland," the pituitary gland is a pea-sized gland located at the base of the brain. It produces and releases several hormones that regulate the function of other endocrine glands, including growth hormone, thyroid-stimulating hormone, adrenocorticotropic hormone, follicle-stimulating hormone, luteinizing hormone, prolactin, and oxytocin.

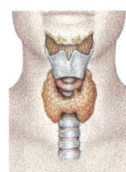

- Thyroid Gland: The thyroid gland is located in the front of the neck and produces hormones such as thyroxine (T4) and triiodothyronine (T3), which regulate metabolism, growth, and energy expenditure.

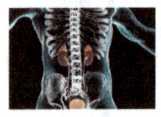

- Adrenal Glands: The adrenal glands are located on top of each kidney and produce hormones such as cortisol (the primary stress hormone), aldosterone (regulates salt and water balance), adrenaline (also known as epinephrine), and noradrenaline (also known as norepinephrine), which regulate the body's response to stress, metabolism, blood pressure, and electrolyte balance.

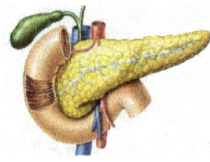

- Pancreas: The pancreas is a dual-function gland located behind the stomach. It produces digestive enzymes that help break down food in the intestine and also secretes hormones such as insulin and glucagon, which regulate blood sugar levels.

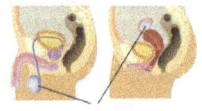

- Gonads: The ovaries in females and testes in males are the primary reproductive glands that produce sex hormones such as estrogen, progesterone, and testosterone, which regulate reproductive function, sexual development, and secondary sexual characteristics.

The endocrine system works in coordination with the nervous system to regulate various physiological processes and maintain overall homeostasis in the body. Dysregulation of hormone production or signaling can lead to endocrine disorders, such as diabetes, thyroid disorders, adrenal insufficiency, and reproductive disorders. Treatment for endocrine disorders often involves hormone replacement therapy, medication, lifestyle modifications, and in some cases, surgical intervention.

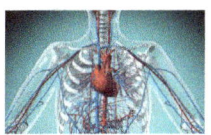

The circulatory system, also known as the cardiovascular system, is a complex network of blood vessels and organs responsible for transporting oxygen, nutrients, hormones, and waste products throughout the body. It plays a crucial role in maintaining homeostasis, delivering essential substances to cells and tissues, removing metabolic waste, and regulating body temperature. *The circulatory system consists of three main components: the heart, blood vessels, and blood.*

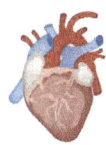

- Heart: The heart is a muscular organ located in the chest cavity between the lungs. It functions as a pump that propels blood throughout the body. The heart is divided into four chambers: the right atrium, right ventricle, left atrium, and left ventricle. Blood enters the heart through the atria and is pumped out through the ventricles to the lungs (pulmonary circulation) for oxygenation and then to the rest of the body (systemic circulation) to deliver oxygen and nutrients.

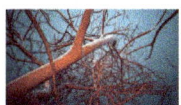

- Blood Vessels: Blood vessels are tubular structures that carry blood throughout the body. There are three main types of blood vessels:

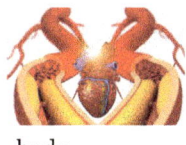

- Arteries: Arteries carry oxygen-rich blood away from the heart to the tissues and organs of the body. The largest artery is the aorta, which originates from the left ventricle of the heart and branches into smaller arteries throughout the body.

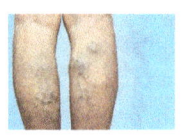
- Veins: Veins carry oxygen-depleted blood back to the heart from the tissues and organs. The largest veins are the superior and inferior vena cava, which return blood to the right atrium of the heart. Veins have one-way valves that prevent backward flow of blood.

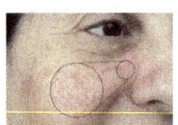
- Capillaries: Capillaries are tiny, thin-walled blood vessels where the exchange of gases, nutrients, and waste products occurs between the blood and surrounding tissues. Capillaries connect arteries to veins and form an extensive network throughout the body.

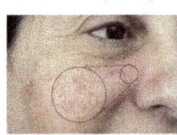
- Blood: Blood is a specialized connective tissue composed of cells suspended in a liquid matrix called plasma. The main components of blood include:

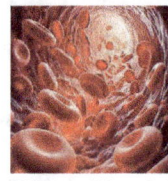
- Red Blood Cells (Erythrocytes): Red blood cells contain hemoglobin, a protein that binds oxygen and carbon dioxide, allowing for the transport of gases between the lungs and tissues.

- White Blood Cells (Leukocytes): White blood cells are involved in the body's immune response and help defend against infection and disease.

- Platelets: Platelets are cell fragments involved in blood clotting and the repair of damaged blood vessels.
- Plasma: Plasma is the liquid portion of blood that carries nutrients, hormones, waste products, and other substances throughout the body.

The circulatory system works in coordination with other organ systems, such as the respiratory system, digestive system, and endocrine system, to maintain overall health and function. Disorders of the circulatory system, such as hypertension, atherosclerosis, heart failure, and stroke, can have serious consequences and may require medical intervention to manage. Maintaining a healthy lifestyle, including regular exercise, a balanced diet, and avoiding tobacco use, can help support cardiovascular health and reduce the risk of circulatory system disorders.

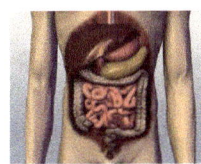
The digestive system is a complex network of organs responsible for the ingestion, digestion, absorption, and elimination of food and waste products from the body. It plays a crucial role in breaking down food into nutrients that can be used by the body for energy, growth, and repair. *The digestive system consists of several organs and structures, each with specific functions:*

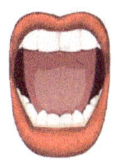
- Mouth: The digestive process begins in the mouth, where food is ingested and mechanically broken down by chewing and mixing with saliva. Saliva contains enzymes, such as amylase, which begin the process of carbohydrate digestion.

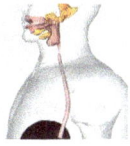
- Esophagus: The esophagus is a muscular tube that connects the mouth to the stomach. It carries chewed food (bolus) from the mouth to the stomach through a series of coordinated muscle contractions called peristalsis.

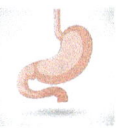
- Stomach: The stomach is a hollow, muscular organ located in the upper abdomen. It serves as a temporary storage reservoir for food and secretes gastric juice, a mixture of hydrochloric acid and enzymes, which breaks down food into a semi-liquid substance called chime.

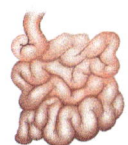
- Small Intestine: The small intestine is the longest part of the digestive tract and consists of three sections: the duodenum, jejunum, and ileum. It plays a critical role in nutrient absorption, as most digestion and absorption of carbohydrates, proteins, fats, vitamins, and minerals occur here. The small intestine is lined with villi and microvilli, tiny finger-like projections that increase the surface area for nutrient absorption.

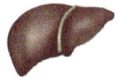
- Liver: The liver is a large organ located in the upper right abdomen. It performs numerous functions, including the

production of bile, which is stored in the gallbladder and released into the small intestine to aid in the digestion and absorption of fats.

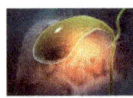
- Gallbladder: The gallbladder is a small, pear-shaped organ located beneath the liver. It stores and concentrates bile produced by the liver and releases it into the small intestine in response to the presence of fatty foods.

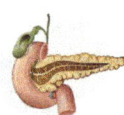
- Pancreas: The pancreas is a glandular organ located behind the stomach. It produces digestive enzymes (such as amylase, lipase, and proteases) and bicarbonate, which are released into the small intestine to aid in the digestion of carbohydrates, fats, and proteins.

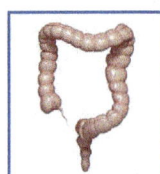
- Large Intestine (Colon): The large intestine is the final portion of the digestive tract and consists of the cecum, colon, rectum, and anus. Its primary functions include reabsorbing water and electrolytes from undigested food, forming and storing feces, and facilitating the elimination of waste products from the body.

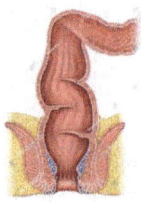
- Rectum and Anus: The rectum is the last part of the large intestine, where feces are stored before elimination. The anus is the opening at the end of the digestive tract through which feces are expelled from the body during defecation.

The digestive system works in coordination with other organ systems, such as the nervous system and endocrine system, to regulate and control digestive processes. Disorders of the digestive system, such as gastro esophageal reflux disease (GERD), irritable bowel syndrome (IBS), inflammatory bowel disease (IBD), and gastrointestinal infections, can cause symptoms such as abdominal pain, bloating, diarrhea, constipation, and malabsorption of nutrients. Maintaining a healthy diet, staying hydrated, and practicing good hygiene and food safety habits can help support digestive health and prevent digestive system disorders.

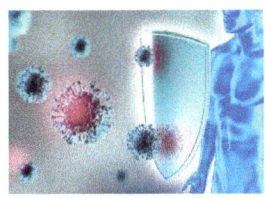 The **immune system** is a complex network of cells, tissues, and organs that work together to defend the body against foreign invaders, such as bacteria, viruses, parasites, and fungi, as well as abnormal cells and substances. Its primary function is to identify and eliminate pathogens while distinguishing them from the body's own healthy cells and tissues. The immune system also plays a crucial role in tissue repair and maintaining overall health and homeostasis. Key components of the *immune system include*:

- White Blood Cells: White blood cells, also known as leukocytes, are specialized immune cells that circulate in the bloodstream and lymphatic system, patrolling the body to detect and destroy pathogens. There are several types of white blood cells, including:

- Neutrophils: Neutrophils are the most abundant type of white blood cells and play a key role in the initial defense against bacterial infections by engulfing and destroying bacteria.

- Lymphocytes: Lymphocytes are a type of white blood cell that includes B cells, T cells, and natural killer (NK) cells. B cells produce antibodies that recognize and neutralize specific pathogens, while T cells regulate immune responses and directly attack infected or abnormal cells. NK cells are responsible for detecting and destroying infected or cancerous cells.

- Monocytes: Monocytes are white blood cells that can differentiate into macrophages and dendritic cells. Macrophages engulf and digest pathogens and debris, while dendritic cells capture and present antigens to activate other immune cells.

- Eosinophil and Basophils: eosinophil and basophils are involved in allergic reactions and defense against parasites.

- Lymphatic System: The lymphatic system is a network of vessels, lymph nodes, and organs (such as the thymus and spleen) that helps maintain fluid balance and filter pathogens and foreign particles from the body. Lymphatic vessels carry lymph, a clear fluid containing white blood cells and waste products, which is filtered through lymph nodes to remove pathogens and activate immune responses.

- Bone Marrow: Bone marrow is the soft, spongy tissue found inside bones, where blood cells, including white blood cells, red blood cells, and platelets, are produced through a process called hematopoiesis.

- Thymus: The thymus is a small gland located in the chest behind the breastbone. It plays a critical role in the maturation and development of T lymphocytes (T cells), which are essential for cell-mediated immunity.
- Spleen: The spleen is a fist-sized organ located in the upper left abdomen. It acts as a blood filter, removing old or damaged red blood cells and pathogens from circulation. The spleen also stores immune cells and plays a role in immune responses to blood-borne pathogens.

- Skin and Mucous Membranes: The skin and mucous membranes lining the respiratory, gastrointestinal, and genitourinary tracts serve as physical barriers that prevent pathogens from entering the body. These surfaces also contain specialized immune cells and produce antimicrobial substances to defend against infections.

- The immune system can be categorized into two main branches:

- Innate Immunity: Innate immunity provides rapid, nonspecific defense against pathogens and is present from birth. It includes physical barriers, such as the skin and mucous membranes, as well as cellular and molecular components, such as neutrophils, macrophages, complement proteins, and antimicrobial peptides.

- Adaptive Immunity: Adaptive immunity is a highly specific and targeted response to specific pathogens and develops over time through exposure to antigens. It involves the activation of B and T lymphocytes, which produce antibodies and coordinate immune responses to eliminate pathogens and provide long-lasting immunity.

The immune system must strike a delicate balance between defending against pathogens and avoiding harmful immune responses against the body's own tissues (autoimmunity) or excessive inflammation (hypersensitivity). Dysregulation of the immune system can lead to immune disorders, such as autoimmune diseases, immunodeficiency disorders, allergies, and inflammatory conditions.

Maintaining a healthy lifestyle, including proper nutrition, regular exercise, adequate sleep, stress management, and vaccination, can help support immune function and reduce the risk of infections and immune-related disorders. Additionally, practicing good hygiene, such as hand washing and avoiding close contact with sick individuals, can help prevent the spread of infectious diseases.

A motion system typically refers to a collection of components and technologies used to control the movement of objects or mechanisms in various applications. These systems are employed in a wide range of fields, including manufacturing, robotics, aerospace, automotive, entertainment, and healthcare. A motion system may involve hardware such as motors, actuators, sensors, and controllers, as well as software for programming and controlling the motion.

Key components of a motion system include:

- Actuators: Devices responsible for converting energy into motion. Examples include electric motors, pneumatic cylinders, hydraulic actuators, piezoelectric actuators, etc.

- Controllers: Devices or systems that manage the operation of actuators and coordinate the motion of different components. Controllers can be simple microcontrollers, programmable logic controllers (PLCs), or more advanced motion controllers.

- Sensors: Devices that provide feedback about the position, velocity, acceleration, force, or other parameters relevant to the motion. Examples include encoders, accelerometers, gyroscopes, proximity sensors, etc.

- Power Transmission Systems: Mechanisms used to transmit power from the actuators to the moving parts. This may involve gears, belts, chains, pulleys, or direct drive systems.
- Software and Programming: Motion systems often require software for programming and configuring motion profiles, coordinating multiple axes of motion, implementing control algorithms, and integrating with higher-level systems.

- Feedback and Control Algorithms: Techniques for analyzing sensor data and implementing control algorithms to regulate the motion accurately, efficiently, and safely. This may involve PID control, trajectory planning, motion profiling, and other control strategies.

Depending on the specific application, a motion system may vary greatly in complexity and performance requirements. Some applications may require high precision, high speed, or synchronization of multiple axes of motion, while others may prioritize energy efficiency, compactness, or robustness in harsh environments.

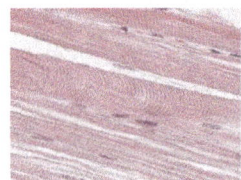

Muscle tissue is one of the four basic types of tissues found in animals, including humans. It is responsible for producing force and causing motion, either within the body (such as the movement of limbs or organs) or externally (such as grasping an object). *There are three main types of muscle tissue:*

- Skeletal Muscle Tissue: Skeletal muscle tissue is attached to bones by tendons and is under voluntary control. It is responsible for movements of the body, such as walking, running, and lifting weights. Skeletal muscle cells, also called muscle fibers, are long, cylindrical, and multinucleated. They contain striations, which are alternating light and dark bands seen under a microscope, due to the arrangement of contractile proteins (actin and myosin). Skeletal muscle contraction is typically fast and powerful.

- Cardiac Muscle Tissue: Cardiac muscle tissue is found exclusively in the heart and is responsible for pumping blood throughout the body. It is striated like skeletal muscle but differs in that it is involuntary and contracts rhythmically without conscious control. Cardiac muscle cells are branched and interconnected, forming a network that allows for coordinated contraction. They are also typically uninucleated. The contraction of cardiac muscle is regulated by specialized cells called pacemaker cells, which generate electrical impulses to coordinate the heartbeat.

- Smooth Muscle Tissue: Smooth muscle tissue is found in the walls of hollow organs, blood vessels, respiratory passageways, and other structures. It is not striated and is typically involuntary, although it can also exhibit some degree of voluntary control in certain situations. Smooth muscle cells are spindle-shaped and contain a single nucleus. Contraction of smooth muscle is slower and more sustained compared to skeletal muscle. It is involved in various physiological processes such as peristalsis (the movement of food through the digestive tract), regulation of blood pressure, and dilation/constriction of blood vessels.

Muscle tissue is highly specialized for its functions and plays a crucial role in maintaining homeostasis and enabling movement and bodily functions.

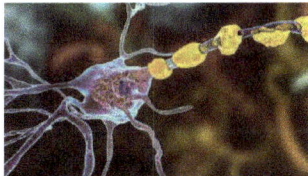

Fat metabolism, also known as lipid metabolism, refers to the biochemical processes involved in the breakdown, synthesis, and utilization of fats (lipids) in the body. It encompasses a complex series of reactions that regulate the storage and release of energy, as well as the maintenance of cellular structure and function.

Here's an overview of the key aspects of fat metabolism:

- Lipolysis: Lipolysis is the process of breaking down stored fats (triglycerides) into fatty acids and glycerol. This occurs primarily in adipose tissue (fat cells) and is stimulated by hormones such as adrenaline and glucagon. Lipolysis is activated during periods of energy deficit, such as fasting or exercise, to provide fatty acids for energy production.

- Fatty Acid Oxidation (Beta-Oxidation): Fatty acids released from adipose tissue or obtained from dietary fats can be oxidized to generate ATP (adenosine triphosphate), the body's primary energy currency. Fatty acid oxidation occurs in the mitochondria of cells, where fatty acids are broken down through a series of enzymatic reactions known as beta-oxidation. This process yields acetyl-CoA molecules, which enter the citric acid cycle (Krebs cycle) to produce ATP through oxidative phosphorylation.

- Ketogenesis: During prolonged fasting or low-carbohydrate diets, the liver converts fatty acids into ketone bodies through a process called ketogenesis. Ketone bodies, such as acetoacetate, beta-hydroxybutyrate, and acetone, serve as alternative fuel sources for tissues like the brain, heart, and skeletal muscles when glucose availability is limited.

- Fat Synthesis (Lipogenesis): Lipogenesis is the process of synthesizing fats from non-lipid precursors, such as glucose or amino acids. This occurs primarily in the liver and adipose tissue and is stimulated by insulin and dietary factors. Excess glucose or calories can be converted into fatty acids and stored as triglycerides in adipose tissue for future energy needs.

- Fat Transport: Fats are transported in the bloodstream as lipoproteins, which are complex particles composed of lipids and proteins. The major lipoproteins involved in fat transport include chylomicrons (transport dietary fats), very-low-density lipoproteins (VLDL), low-density lipoproteins (LDL), and high-density lipoproteins (HDL). These lipoproteins facilitate the transport of lipids to and from various tissues in the body.

- Regulation: Fat metabolism is tightly regulated by hormonal signals, nutritional status, and metabolic demands. Hormones such as insulin, glucagon, adrenaline (epinephrine), and leptin play key roles in modulating lipid metabolism by regulating processes like lipolysis, lipogenesis, and fatty acid oxidation.

Overall, fat metabolism is essential for energy production, maintaining metabolic homeostasis and providing structural components for cell membranes and signaling molecules. Dysregulation of lipid metabolism can contribute to metabolic disorders such as obesity, diabetes, and cardiovascular disease.

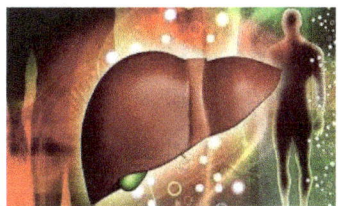
Detoxification refers to the body's process of neutralizing, transforming, or eliminating potentially harmful substances, including toxins, drugs, and metabolic waste products. These substances may be generated internally as byproducts of normal metabolic processes or acquired from the external environment through ingestion, inhalation, or absorption.

Detoxification primarily occurs in the liver, although other organs such as the kidneys, lungs, skin, and intestines also play important roles in eliminating toxins. The liver contains specialized enzymes and biochemical pathways that facilitate the detoxification process, *including:*

- Phase I Detoxification: Involves enzymatic reactions (e.g., oxidation, reduction, hydrolysis) that convert lipophilic (fat-soluble) toxins into more water-soluble intermediates, making them easier to eliminate from the body.

- Phase II Detoxification: Involves conjugation reactions, where water-soluble molecules (e.g., glutathione, sulfate, glucuronic acid) are added to Phase I metabolites to further enhance their solubility and facilitate excretion.
- Excretion: Once detoxified, the water-soluble metabolites are typically excreted from the body via urine, feces, sweat, or exhalation.

Metabolism:

Metabolism encompasses all the biochemical processes that occur within cells to maintain life. It involves the conversion of nutrients (e.g., carbohydrates, fats, proteins) into energy and building blocks for cellular components, as well as the synthesis and breakdown of molecules necessary for various physiological functions.

Key aspects of metabolism include:

- Catabolism: The breakdown of complex molecules into simpler ones, usually accompanied by the release of energy. For example, carbohydrates, fats, and proteins are broken down through processes such as glycolysis, beta-oxidation, and proteolysis to produce ATP, the body's primary energy currency.

- Anabolism: The synthesis of complex molecules from simpler ones, typically requiring energy input. Examples include the synthesis of proteins, carbohydrates, and lipids for cellular growth, repair, and maintenance.

- Energy Production: Metabolism involves the conversion of nutrients into energy (ATP) through processes such as cellular respiration (oxidative phosphorylation) and fermentation (in the absence of oxygen).

Relationship between Detoxification and Metabolism:

Detoxification processes in the liver often involve metabolic reactions mediated by enzymes and co-factors. For example, many detoxification enzymes involved in Phase I and Phase II reactions are part of the liver's metabolic pathways.

Metabolism provides the energy and molecular building blocks necessary for detoxification processes to occur. ATP generated through metabolism is required for various detoxification reactions, and metabolic intermediates may serve as substrates or co-factors for detoxification enzymes.

Conversely, detoxification helps to eliminate potentially harmful byproducts of metabolism, such as reactive oxygen species (ROS) and toxic metabolites, thereby protecting cells and tissues from damage.

In summary, while detoxification and metabolism are distinct processes with specific functions, they are closely intertwined and mutually supportive in maintaining the body's overall health and function. Proper regulation and coordination of these processes are essential for optimal physiological functioning and the body's ability to adapt to internal and external challenges.

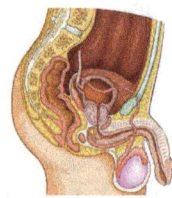
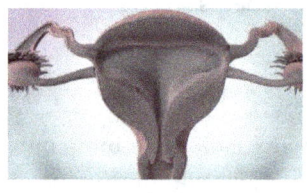

The reproductive system, also known as the genital system, is a collection of organs and tissues in organisms responsible for reproduction. Its primary function is to produce offspring, ensuring the continuation of a species. In humans, the reproductive system consists of both internal and external organs, as well as hormonal and neurological control systems. Here's an overview of the main components and functions of the human reproductive system:

Primary Reproductive Organs:

Male Reproductive System:

- Testes: Male gonads that produce sperm and testosterone.
- Epididymis: A coiled tube where sperm mature and are stored.
- Vas deferens: A duct that carries sperm from the epididymis to the urethra during ejaculation.
- Seminal vesicles, prostate gland, and bulbourethral glands: Glands that produce seminal fluid, which nourishes and transports sperm during ejaculation.
- Penis: Male organ used for sexual intercourse and ejaculation.

Female Reproductive System:

- Ovaries: Female gonads that produce eggs (ova) and sex hormones, including estrogen and progesterone.
- Fallopian tubes (oviducts): Tubes that transport eggs from the ovaries to the uterus. Fertilization typically occurs in the fallopian tubes.
- Uterus (womb): A hollow, muscular organ where a fertilized egg implants and develops into a fetus during pregnancy.
- Cervix: The lower part of the uterus that connects to the vagina.
- Vagina: A muscular canal that serves as the birth canal during childbirth and also receives sperm during sexual intercourse.

Accessory Reproductive Organs:

- Male Accessory Organs: These include the seminal vesicles, prostate gland, and bulbourethral glands, which produce seminal fluid that mixes with sperm to form semen.

- Female Accessory Organs: These include the mammary glands (breasts), which produce milk to nourish newborns during lactation.

Hormonal Control:

The reproductive system is regulated by hormones produced by the hypothalamus, pituitary gland, and gonads (testes in males, ovaries in females).

In males, the hypothalamus releases gonadotropin-releasing hormone (GnRH), which stimulates the pituitary gland to release luteinizing hormone (LH) and follicle-stimulating hormone (FSH). LH and FSH act on the testes to regulate sperm production and testosterone secretion.

In females, the hypothalamus and pituitary gland regulate the menstrual cycle and ovulation by releasing GnRH, LH, and FSH. These hormones stimulate the ovaries to produce estrogen and progesterone, which regulate the menstrual cycle and prepare the uterus for pregnancy.

Gametogenesis:

Gametogenesis is the process of producing gametes (sperm and eggs) through meiosis.

In males, spermatogenesis occurs in the testes and produces sperm cells.

In females, oogenesis occurs in the ovaries and produces egg cells (ova).

Fertilization and Pregnancy:

Fertilization occurs when a sperm cell fertilizes an egg cell, resulting in the formation of a zygote.

The zygote undergoes cleavage and implantation in the uterus, leading to pregnancy.

During pregnancy, the developing fetus receives nutrients and oxygen from the mother's bloodstream through the placenta.

Overall, the reproductive system is essential for the perpetuation of life and involves complex interactions between organs, hormones, and physiological processes. Its functions include the production of gametes, fertilization, pregnancy, childbirth, and lactation, all of which are crucial for the survival and continuation of species.

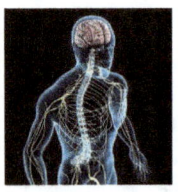

The nervous system is a complex network of specialized cells, tissues, and organs that coordinate and regulate the activities of the body. It is divided into two main parts: the central nervous system (CNS) and the peripheral nervous system (PNS). *Here's an overview of each*:

- Central Nervous System (CNS):

The CNS consists of the brain and spinal cord.

- Brain: The brain is the control center of the nervous system and the body. It is responsible for processing sensory information, initiating responses, regulating body functions, and coordinating complex behaviors and actions. The brain is divided into several regions, each with specific functions, including the cerebrum, cerebellum, brainstem, and diencephalon.

- Spinal Cord: The spinal cord is a long, tubular structure that extends from the base of the brain down the vertebral column. It serves as a relay system between the brain and the rest of the body, transmitting sensory information from the PNS to the brain and motor commands from the brain to the muscles and glands.

Peripheral Nervous System (PNS):

The PNS includes all nervous tissue outside the CNS.

- Sensory Division: The sensory division of the PNS is responsible for detecting sensory stimuli from the external environment and internal body systems. It consists of sensory receptors (such as those for touch, temperature, pain, and proprioception) and sensory neurons that transmit this information to the CNS.

- Motor Division: The motor division of the PNS controls voluntary and involuntary movements and actions. It consists of motor neurons that carry signals from the CNS to muscles and glands.

- Somatic Nervous System: The somatic nervous system controls voluntary movements of skeletal muscles and receives sensory input from the external environment.
- Autonomic Nervous System (ANS): The ANS regulates involuntary functions of internal organs and glands. It is further divided into the sympathetic nervous system (which mobilizes the body's fight-or-flight response) and the parasympathetic nervous system (which promotes rest, relaxation, and digestion).

Neurons:

Neurons are the basic functional units of the nervous system. They are specialized cells capable of transmitting electrical impulses (action potentials) and chemical signals (neurotransmitters) to communicate with other neurons and target cells.

Neurons consist of three main parts: dendrites (which receive signals from other neurons), a cell body (which contains the nucleus and organelles), and an axon (which transmits signals to other neurons or target cells).

Neurons communicate with each other and with target cells (such as muscles and glands) through synapses, specialized junctions where neurotransmitters are released from the presynaptic neuron and bind to receptors on the postsynaptic cell.

Supporting Cells:

Supporting cells in the nervous system provide structural support, insulation, and metabolic support to neurons.

Glial cells, including astrocytes, oligodendrocytes, Schwann cells, and microglia, perform various functions such as maintaining the blood-brain barrier, myelinating axons, and modulating synaptic transmission.

Glial cells play crucial roles in neural development, plasticity, and repair.

Overall, the nervous system is essential for coordinating and regulating sensory perception, motor responses, cognitive functions, and homeostasis in the body. It allows organisms to interact with their environment, respond to stimuli, and adapt to changing conditions, ensuring their survival and well-being.

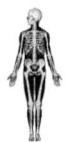 **The human skeleton** is the internal framework of bones that provides structure, support, and protection for the body's soft tissues and organs. It also serves as an attachment site for muscles, facilitates movement, and plays a crucial role in mineral storage and blood cell production. *Here's an overview of the human skeleton*:

- Composition:

The human skeleton is composed of approximately 206 bones, although this number can vary slightly from person to person due to individual differences, particularly in the small bones of the hands and feet.

Bones are classified into two main types: axial skeleton and appendicular skeleton.

- Axial Skeleton:

The axial skeleton consists of the bones along the body's central axis, including the skull, vertebral column, and rib cage.

- Skull: The skull is composed of cranial bones (which encase and protect the brain) and facial bones (which form the structure of the face). It includes the cranium, mandible (lower jaw), maxilla (upper jaw), nasal bones, and various other bones.

- Vertebral Column: The vertebral column, or spine, is composed of individual vertebrae separated by intervertebral discs. It provides support for the body, protects the spinal cord, and allows for flexibility and movement. The vertebral column is divided into five regions: cervical, thoracic, lumbar, sacral, and coccygeal.

- Rib Cage: The rib cage consists of the ribs, sternum (breastbone), and thoracic vertebrae. It encloses and protects the heart, lungs, and other vital organs in the thoracic cavity.

Appendicular Skeleton:

The appendicular skeleton consists of the bones of the limbs (arms and legs) and their associated girdles (shoulder girdle and pelvic girdle).

- Shoulder Girdle: The shoulder girdle includes the clavicle (collarbone) and scapula (shoulder blade). It attaches the upper limbs to the axial skeleton.

- Upper Limbs: Each upper limb consists of the humerus (upper arm bone), radius and ulna (forearm bones), carpals (wrist bones), metacarpals (palm bones), and phalanges (finger bones).

- Pelvic Girdle: The pelvic girdle consists of two hip bones (coxal bones) that articulate with the sacrum at the sacroiliac joints. It supports the trunk of the body and provides attachment for the lower limbs.

- Lower Limbs: Each lower limb consists of the femur (thigh bone), patella (kneecap), tibia and fibula (lower leg bones), tarsals (ankle bones), metatarsals (foot bones), and phalanges (toe bones).

Functions:

- Support: The skeleton provides a rigid framework that supports and maintains the shape of the body.

- Protection: Bones protect vital organs such as the brain, heart, and lungs from injury.

- Movement: Muscles attached to bones by tendons pull on them to produce movement at joints.

- Mineral Storage: Bones store minerals such as calcium and phosphorus, which are important for bone strength and metabolic functions.

- Hematopoiesis: Certain bones contain red bone marrow, where blood cells (red blood cells, white blood cells, and platelets) are produced through a process called hematopoiesis.

Overall, the human skeleton is a complex and dynamic structure that is essential for various physiological functions, including support, protection, movement, and mineral storage.

CHANNELS AND CHOLETERALS

The Hand Tai Yin Lung Meridian is one of the twelve primary meridians in traditional Chinese medicine (TCM). Meridians are channels or pathways through which qi (vital energy) flows throughout the body. Each meridian is associated with specific organs and functions, and they are an integral part of acupuncture and other TCM practices. Here's an overview of the Hand Tai Yin Lung Meridian:

Location:

- The Hand Tai Yin Lung Meridian originates from the lateral aspect of the chest, just below the clavicle (collarbone), near the first rib.

- It runs downward and inward along the anterior aspect of the upper arm, passing through the cubital fossa (elbow crease).

From there, it continues down the medial aspect of the forearm, passing through the wrist and ending at the radial side of the tip of the thumb.

Associated Organ and Function:

The Hand Tai Yin Lung Meridian is associated with the lungs, which are responsible for respiration and the exchange of oxygen and carbon dioxide in the body.

In TCM, the lungs are also believed to govern qi and regulate the circulation of qi and fluids throughout the body. They are associated with the skin, the body's first line of defense against external pathogens.

- Acupuncture Points:

The Hand Tai Yin Lung Meridian has nine acupuncture points along its pathway. These points can be stimulated with acupuncture needles, acupressure, or other therapeutic techniques to regulate the flow of qi and treat various health conditions.

Some of the major acupuncture points on the Hand Tai Yin Lung Meridian include Lung 1 (Zhong Fu), Lung 5 (Chi Ze), Lung 9 (Tai Yuan), and Lung 11 (Shao Shang). Each point has specific indications and therapeutic effects according to TCM theory.

- Clinical Applications:

The Hand Tai Yin Lung Meridian is commonly used in TCM clinical practice to treat respiratory disorders such as asthma, cough, bronchitis, and pneumonia.

It is also utilized for conditions related to the skin, such as eczema, itching, and other dermatological issues.

Additionally, acupuncture along this meridian may be employed to regulate qi and relieve emotional imbalances, as the lungs are associated with grief and sadness in TCM theory.

- Energetic Qualities:

In TCM, the Hand Tai Yin Lung Meridian is considered yin in nature and is associated with qualities such as receptivity, nourishment, and introspection.

Imbalances in the Lung Meridian, such as stagnation or deficiency of qi, can manifest as respiratory symptoms, skin disorders, or emotional disturbances.

Overall, the Hand Tai Yin Lung Meridian plays a significant role in regulating respiratory function, supporting the immune system, and maintaining overall health and vitality according to traditional Chinese medicine principles.

The Hand Yang Ming Large Intestine Meridian is one of the twelve primary meridians in traditional Chinese medicine (TCM). Meridians are pathways through which qi (vital energy) flows throughout the body. Each meridian is associated with specific organs and functions and is utilized in acupuncture, acupressure, and other TCM modalities. Here's an overview of the Hand Yangming Large Intestine Meridian:

- Location:

The Hand Yang Ming Large Intestine Meridian starts at the tip of the index finger.

From there, it runs along the radial side (thumb side) of the hand, along the dorsum of the hand and the wrist.

It continues up the lateral aspect of the forearm, passing through the elbow crease (cubital fossa).

Finally, it travels up the lateral aspect of the upper arm and ends at the lateral aspect of the nostril.

- Associated Organ and Function:

The Hand Yang Ming Large Intestine Meridian is associated with the large intestine, which is responsible for the final stages of digestion and the elimination of waste products from the body.

In TCM, the large intestine is also believed to play a role in the regulation of water metabolism and the transformation of waste material into feces.

- Acupuncture Points:

The Hand Yang Ming Large Intestine Meridian has twenty points along its pathway, including its starting point at the tip of the index finger.

Some major acupuncture points on the Hand Yang Ming Large Intestine Meridian include Large Intestine 4 (Hegu), Large Intestine 11 (Quchi), and Large Intestine 20 (Xinxiang). Each point has specific indications and therapeutic effects according to TCM theory.

- Clinical Applications:

The Hand Yang Ming Large Intestine Meridian is commonly used in TCM clinical practice to treat disorders of the large intestine and related conditions.

Acupuncture along this meridian may be employed to alleviate symptoms such as constipation, diarrhea, abdominal pain, bloating, and other digestive issues.

It is also utilized for conditions affecting the head and face, such as sinusitis, nasal congestion, toothache, and headaches.

- Energetic Qualities:

In TCM, the Hand Yang Ming Large Intestine Meridian is considered yang in nature and is associated with qualities such as activity, movement, and elimination.

Imbalances in the Large Intestine Meridian, such as stagnation or excess heat, can manifest as digestive disturbances, headaches, or other symptoms related to the large intestine and associated organs.

Overall, the Hand Yang Ming Large Intestine Meridian is an important pathway in TCM theory, utilized to regulate digestive function, relieve pain, and promote overall health and balance within the body

In traditional Chinese medicine (TCM), there is a concept of dietary therapy that involves selecting foods based on their energetic properties to support and balance the body's organ systems, including the meridians. The Tai Yin Lung Meridian is one of the twelve primary meridians in TCM, and according to TCM theory, certain foods can be beneficial for nourishing and supporting the Lung Meridian. These foods are believed to have properties that resonate with the energetic characteristics of the Lung Meridian and may help promote its health and function. *Here are some dietary recommendations for the Tai Yin Lung Meridian:*

- Pungent Foods:

Pungent flavors are said to have an affinity for the Lung Meridian and can help stimulate lung function and disperse excess phlegm.

Examples of pungent foods include onions, garlic, ginger, radishes, mustard greens, and peppers.

- White-Colored Foods:

In TCM, the Lung Meridian is associated with the color white, and consuming white-colored foods is believed to nourish and support this meridian.

Examples of white-colored foods include white rice, cauliflower, daikon radish, white beans, tofu, and white mushrooms.

- Moistening Foods:

The Lung Meridian is associated with the element of Metal, which is related to dryness. Consuming moistening foods can help counteract dryness and support lung health.

Moistening foods include pears, apples, bananas, honey, spinach, cucumber, and melons.

- Aromatic Herbs and Spices:

Aromatic herbs and spices are often used in TCM to promote circulation, stimulate digestion, and support respiratory health.

Examples include cinnamon, fennel, cardamom, mint, basil, and thyme.

- Hydration:

Adequate hydration is essential for maintaining healthy lung function and preventing dryness. Drinking plenty of water and consuming hydrating foods such as soups, broths, and watery fruits and vegetables can support lung health.

- Avoiding Excessive Dairy and Cold Foods:

In TCM, excessive consumption of cold or dairy-based foods is believed to weaken the lungs and contribute to phlegm accumulation. Limiting or avoiding these foods may be beneficial for supporting lung health.

It's important to note that individual dietary recommendations may vary based on factors such as constitution, underlying health conditions, and seasonal considerations. Consulting with a qualified TCM practitioner or healthcare provider can help tailor dietary recommendations to individual needs and goals. Additionally, incorporating a variety of nutrient-dense foods and maintaining a balanced diet is important for overall health and well-being.

The Hand Shao Yin Heart Meridian often referred to as the Heart Meridian in traditional Chinese medicine (TCM), is one of the twelve primary meridians in the body. Meridians are pathways through which qi (vital energy) flows, and each meridian is associated with specific organs and functions. The Heart Meridian is considered crucial for regulating blood circulation, housing the spirit (shen), and influencing emotional well-being according to TCM principles.

The Heart Sutra, on the other hand, is a Buddhist scripture that is highly revered in Mahayana Buddhism, particularly in the Zen and Tibetan traditions. It is a concise text that encapsulates the teachings of emptiness (shunyata) and wisdom in Buddhism. While it is not directly related to TCM or the Heart Meridian, the concept of the heart in Buddhism can be metaphorically linked to the Heart Meridian's role in TCM.

In TCM, the Heart Meridian is believed to govern various physiological and psychological functions, *including:*

- Circulation: The Heart Meridian is associated with regulating blood circulation and ensuring the smooth flow of blood throughout the body. Any imbalance in the Heart Meridian may manifest as circulatory issues such as poor circulation, palpitations, or blood stasis.

- Emotions and Mental Health: The Heart Meridian is closely linked to the concept of the shen, which encompasses the mind, spirit, and consciousness in TCM. It is believed to influence emotional well-being, mental clarity, and consciousness. Imbalances in the Heart Meridian may manifest as emotional disturbances such as anxiety, insomnia, or depression.

- Connection to Other Organs: According to TCM theory, the Heart Meridian is interconnected with other organs and meridians in the body, including the Small Intestine Meridian, Pericardium Meridian, and Triple Burner Meridian. These connections are believed to play a role in maintaining overall balance and harmony within the body.

In summary, while there is no direct correlation between the Heart Sutra and the Heart Meridian in TCM, both concepts share symbolic significance related to the heart, consciousness, and well-being. The Heart Meridian's role in TCM encompasses physiological functions such as blood circulation and emotional regulation, while the Heart Sutra conveys profound teachings on wisdom and emptiness in Buddhism.

Hand Tai Yang Small Intestine Meridian" in traditional Chinese medicine (TCM). Meridians are pathways through which qi (vital energy) flows in the body, and each meridian is associated with specific organs and functions. The Small Intestine Meridian is one of the twelve primary meridians in TCM, and it is connected to the Tai Yang aspect of the body, which relates to the energetic qualities of the sun.

Here's an overview of the Hand Tai Yang Small Intestine Meridian:

- Location:

The Hand Tai Yang Small Intestine Meridian starts at the ulnar side (pinky finger side) of the tip of the little finger.

It travels along the posterior aspect (back) of the arm, passing through the back of the shoulder and the scapula (shoulder blade).

From there, it continues down the back of the trunk, running along the lateral side of the spine.

- The meridian then splits into two branches:

One branch continues up to the neck and passes through the jaw, cheekbone, and ear.

The other branch travels across the scapula and ends at the shoulder.

- Associated Organ and Function:

The Small Intestine Meridian is associated with the small intestine organ, which plays a crucial role in the digestion and absorption of nutrients from food.

In TCM, the Small Intestine Meridian is believed to regulate the flow of fluids and nutrients in the body, as well as separate the clear from the turbid.

- Acupuncture Points:

The Hand Tai Yang Small Intestine Meridian has nineteen acupuncture points along its pathway.

Some major acupuncture points on the Small Intestine Meridian include Small Intestine 3 (Houxi), Small Intestine 6 (Yanglao), and Small Intestine 11 (Tianzong).

- Clinical Applications:

Acupuncture along the Small Intestine Meridian is used in TCM clinical practice to treat various conditions related to the small intestine and adjacent areas.

It may be employed to alleviate symptoms such as abdominal pain, bloating, diarrhea, constipation, and digestive disturbances.

- Energetic Qualities:

The Hand Tai Yang Small Intestine Meridian is considered yang in nature, and it is associated with qualities such as activity, movement, and transformation.

Imbalances in the Small Intestine Meridian may manifest as digestive issues, discomfort along the pathway of the meridian, or emotional disturbances related to the small intestine's functions.

Overall, the Hand Tai Yang Small Intestine Meridian is an important pathway in TCM theory, utilized to regulate digestion, promote the flow of fluids and nutrients, and maintain overall balance and harmony within the body.

The Foot Tai Yang Bladder Meridian is one of the twelve primary meridians in traditional Chinese medicine (TCM). Meridians are pathways through which qi (vital energy) flows in the body, and each meridian is associated with specific organs and functions. The Bladder Meridian is significant in TCM for its role in regulating the flow of bodily fluids, supporting urinary function, and influencing various physiological processes. *Here's an overview of the Foot Tai Yang Bladder Meridian:*

- Location:

The Foot Tai Yang Bladder Meridian starts from the inner corner of the eye (near the tear duct) and runs along the side of the head and neck.

It travels down the back of the body, following a zigzag pattern along the paravertebral muscles (located on either side of the spine) on the back.

From the neck, it descends along the upper back, lower back, buttocks, and back of the legs.

The meridian then splits into two branches:

One branch continues down the back of the leg, passing through the back of the knee and ankle.

The other branch extends to the lateral side of the foot, ending at the outside edge of the small toe.

- Associated Organ and Function:

The Bladder Meridian is associated with the bladder organ, which is responsible for storing and eliminating urine from the body.

In TCM, the Bladder Meridian is believed to regulate the flow of qi and bodily fluids, support urinary function, and influence the water metabolism in the body.

- Acupuncture Points:

The Foot Tai Yang Bladder Meridian has sixty-seven acupuncture points along its pathway, making it one of the meridians with the most acupuncture points.

Some major acupuncture points on the Bladder Meridian include Bladder 1 (Jingling), Bladder 10 (Tianzhu), Bladder 23 (Shenshu), and Bladder 40 (Weizhong).

- Clinical Applications:

Acupuncture along the Bladder Meridian is used in TCM clinical practice to treat various conditions related to the bladder, back, and adjacent areas.

It may be employed to alleviate symptoms such as urinary dysfunction, back pain, sciatica, muscle tension, and other issues affecting the pathway of the meridian.

- Energetic Qualities:

The Foot Tai Yang Bladder Meridian is considered yang in nature and is associated with qualities such as strength, resilience, and endurance.

Imbalances in the Bladder Meridian may manifest as urinary problems, back pain, stiffness along the back of the body, or emotional disturbances related to water metabolism and the bladder's functions.

Overall, the Foot Tai Yang Bladder Meridian is an essential pathway in TCM theory, utilized to regulate urinary function, promote the flow of qi and bodily fluids, and maintain overall balance and harmony within the body.

The Foot Jue Yin Liver Meridian is one of the twelve primary meridians in traditional Chinese medicine (TCM). Meridians are pathways through which qi (vital energy) flows in the body, and each meridian is associated with specific organs and functions. The Liver Meridian is significant in TCM for its role in regulating the flow of qi, supporting liver function, and influencing various physiological processes. Here's an overview of the Foot Jue Yin Liver Meridian:

- Location:

The Foot Jue Yin Liver Meridian starts at the lateral side of the big toe.

It travels upward along the top of the foot, running between the first and second toes.

From there, it ascends along the inner aspect of the lower leg, passing through the medial aspect of the knee.

The meridian then continues upward along the inner thigh and abdomen, passing through the groin area.

It travels internally through the liver, diaphragm, and lungs, eventually connecting with the pericardium and heart meridians.

- Associated Organ and Function:

The Liver Meridian is associated with the liver organ, which plays a vital role in detoxification, metabolism, and the regulation of various physiological processes.

In TCM, the Liver Meridian is believed to regulate the smooth flow of qi throughout the body, maintain the balance of emotions, and support the free movement of blood and qi.

- Acupuncture Points:

The Foot Jue Yin Liver Meridian has fourteen acupuncture points along its pathway.

Some major acupuncture points on the Liver Meridian include Liver 3 (Taichung), Liver 8 (Ququan), Liver 13 (Zhangmen), and Liver 14 (Qi men).

- Clinical Applications:

Acupuncture along the Liver Meridian is used in TCM clinical practice to treat various conditions related to the liver, digestive system, and emotional well-being.

It may be employed to alleviate symptoms such as liver dysfunction, digestive disturbances, menstrual disorders, emotional imbalances, and musculoskeletal pain along the pathway of the meridian.

- Energetic Qualities:

The Foot Jue Yin Liver Meridian is considered yin in nature and is associated with qualities such as nourishment, receptivity, and emotional balance.

Imbalances in the Liver Meridian may manifest as liver stagnation, emotional disturbances (such as irritability or depression), digestive issues, menstrual irregularities, or musculoskeletal pain along the pathway of the meridian.

Overall, the Foot Jue Yin Liver Meridian is an important pathway in TCM theory, utilized to regulate liver function, promote the smooth flow of qi and blood, and maintain overall balance and harmony within the body.

The Ren Channel, also known as the Ren Mai or Conception Vessel, is one of the eight extraordinary meridians in traditional Chinese medicine (TCM). Unlike the twelve primary meridians, which are bilateral and associated with specific organs, the extraordinary meridians are unpaired and have unique functions in regulating the flow of qi (vital energy) and blood throughout the body. Here's an overview of the Ren Channel:

- Location:

The Ren Channel runs along the anterior midline of the body.

It originates in the lower abdomen, below the navel (around the pubic region), and ascends along the midline of the abdomen, chest, and throat.

The Ren Channel terminates at the chin, where it connects with the conception vessel points on the face.

Associated Organs and Functions:

The Ren Channel is associated with the yin aspect of the body and is believed to regulate the functions of the yin organs (such as the heart, lungs, spleen, liver, and kidneys).

It plays a role in regulating the circulation of qi and blood in the abdomen, chest, and throat regions.

The Ren Channel is also associated with reproduction, menstruation, and the nourishment of the fetus during pregnancy.

Acupuncture Points:

The Ren Channel has twenty-four acupuncture points along its pathway.

Some major acupuncture points on the Ren Channel include Ren 1 (Huiyin), Ren 4 (Guanyuan), Ren 6 (Qihai), Ren 12 (Zhongwan), Ren 17 (Shanzhong), and Ren 22 (Tiantu).

- Clinical Applications:

Acupuncture along the Ren Channel is used in TCM clinical practice to treat various conditions related to the abdomen, chest, throat, and reproductive system.

It may be employed to alleviate symptoms such as abdominal pain, bloating, chest congestion, throat disorders, menstrual irregularities, infertility, and pregnancy-related issues.

- Energetic Qualities:

The Ren Channel is considered a major pathway for the circulation of yin energy in the body.

It is associated with qualities such as nourishment, receptivity, and the regulation of internal functions.

Imbalances in the Ren Channel may manifest as symptoms related to dysfunction in the yin organs, reproductive system, or emotional disturbances associated with yin energy.

Overall, the Ren Channel plays a vital role in regulating the circulation of yin energy, nourishing the body's internal organs, and supporting reproductive health according to TCM principles. Acupuncture and other TCM modalities are used to balance and harmonize the flow of qi and blood through the Ren Channel, promoting overall health and well-being.

The Governor Meridian, also known as the Du Mai or Governing Vessel, is one of the eight extraordinary meridians in traditional Chinese medicine (TCM). Unlike the twelve primary meridians, which are bilateral and associated with specific organs, the extraordinary meridians have unique functions in regulating the flow of qi (vital energy) and blood throughout the body. Here's an overview of the Governor Meridian:

- Location:

The Governor Meridian runs along the midline of the body, parallel to the spine.

It originates at the perineum, near the tip of the coccyx (tailbone), and ascends along the spine.

From there, it travels up the back of the head and neck, crossing over the crown of the head, and terminates at the upper lip.

- Function:

The Governor Meridian is responsible for regulating the flow of qi and controlling the distribution of qi throughout the body.

It serves as a major pathway for the circulation of yang energy in the body, helping to maintain balance between yin and yang.

The Governor Meridian also plays a role in supporting the function of the spine, brain, and central nervous system.

- Acupuncture Points:

The Governor Meridian has twenty-seven acupuncture points along its pathway.

Some major acupuncture points on the Governor Meridian include Du 1 (Changqiang), Du 4 (Mingmen), Du 14 (Dazhui), Du 20 (Baihui), and Du 26 (Shuigou).

- Clinical Applications:

Acupuncture along the Governor Meridian is used in TCM clinical practice to treat various conditions related to the spine, brain, central nervous system, and overall energy balance.

It may be employed to alleviate symptoms such as back pain, neck stiffness, headaches, dizziness, insomnia, and emotional imbalances.

The Governor Meridian is also utilized for enhancing mental clarity, concentration, and spiritual development in TCM and martial arts practices.

- Energetic Qualities:

The Governor Meridian is associated with yang energy and is believed to govern the upward flow of qi in the body.

It is considered a major pathway for the circulation of yang energy and the regulation of vital functions.

Imbalances in the Governor Meridian may manifest as symptoms related to dysfunction in the spine, brain, or nervous system, as well as disturbances in the flow of yang energy.

Overall, the Governor Meridian plays a vital role in regulating the flow of qi and supporting the function of the spine, brain, and central nervous system. Acupuncture and other TCM modalities are used to balance and harmonize the flow of qi through the Governor Meridian, promoting overall health and well-being.

Qi is central to TCM theory, and meridians are pathways through which qi flows in the body. Each meridian is associated with specific organs and functions, contributing to the overall balance and harmony of qi in the body.

While there isn't a meridian specifically named the "vital meridian," the concept of vitality and the regulation of qi flow are integral to TCM practice. Practitioners work to balance and harmonize the flow of qi through the meridians to support overall health and well-being. This may involve assessing and treating imbalances in the individual meridians or addressing underlying disharmonies in the body's energy system as a whole.

If you have a specific question or topic related to TCM and meridians, feel free to provide more details, and I'd be happy to offer further information or assistance!

Dai Channel," which is also known as the "Girdling Vessel" or "Belt Vessel" in traditional Chinese medicine (TCM). The Dai Mai is considered one of the eight extraordinary meridians in TCM, and it plays a unique role in regulating the flow of qi (vital energy) throughout the body. *Here's an overview of the Dai Mai:*

- Location:

The Dai Mai runs horizontally around the waist, encircling the body like a belt.

It doesn't follow a linear pathway like the primary meridians but rather wraps around the waistline.

- Function:

The Dai Mai is responsible for connecting the six yang meridians of the arms and legs, namely the Triple Burner, Gallbladder, Stomach, Small Intestine, Large Intestine, and Bladder meridians.

It helps to regulate the balance between yin and yang energy in the body and supports the proper distribution of qi among the yang meridians.

The Dai Mai also plays a role in stabilizing the lower back and pelvis, providing structural support to the body.

- Clinical Applications:

Imbalances in the Dai Mai can manifest as symptoms such as lower back pain, hip pain, sciatica, digestive issues, and emotional instability.

Treatment of the Dai Mai involves techniques aimed at restoring balance and harmony to the flow of qi around the waistline, such as acupuncture, acupressure, moxibustion, and qigong exercises.

- Energetic Qualities:

The Dai Mai is associated with the Wood element in TCM theory, and it is closely related to the concept of the liver's function in regulating the smooth flow of qi.

Imbalances in the Dai Mai may reflect disturbances in the liver's function and the proper distribution of qi in the body.

Overall, the Dai Mai plays a significant role in regulating the flow of qi among the six yang meridians of the arms and legs and supporting the structural integrity of the lower back and pelvis. Balancing the Dai Mai is essential for maintaining overall health and well-being in TCM practice.

PULSE OF HEART AND BRAIN

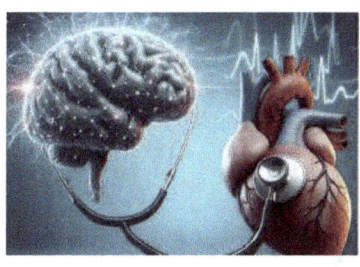

In the context of human health, particularly cardiovascular health, the term "stroke index" refers to a parameter used in hemodynamics to assess the efficiency of the heart's pumping function. It is a measure of the amount of blood ejected from the heart with each heartbeat, adjusted for body surface area. The stroke index is calculated by dividing the cardiac output (the volume of blood pumped by the heart per minute) by the body surface area.

The stroke index is expressed in units of volume per unit area (e.g., milliliters per square meter) and is used to evaluate cardiac function and hemodynamic status. It provides information about the heart's ability to pump blood effectively relative to the size of the individual.

A normal stroke index typically falls within a specific range, which may vary depending on factors such as age, gender, and overall health status. Deviations from the normal range may indicate underlying cardiovascular issues or changes in hemodynamic status that require further evaluation and management.

Monitoring the stroke index can be helpful in various clinical settings, including critical care, cardiology, and perioperative care, to assess cardiac function, guide treatment decisions, and evaluate the response to interventions aimed at optimizing cardiovascular health.

Stroke volume refers to the amount of blood ejected by the heart's left ventricle with each contraction, or heartbeat. It's an essential parameter used to assess cardiac function and overall cardiovascular health. Stroke volume is typically measured in milliliters (ml) and is influenced by various factors, including heart rate, preload, afterload, and contractility.

Here's a breakdown of stroke volume and its significance in human physiology:

- Measurement: Stroke volume is often measured using various techniques, including echocardiography (ultrasound imaging of the heart), cardiac catheterization, and impedance cardiography. These methods allow healthcare providers to accurately assess the volume of blood pumped out of the left ventricle per beat.

- Formula: Stroke volume can be calculated using the formula:

- Stroke Volume = End-Diastolic Volume - End-Systolic Volume
- Where:
- End-Diastolic Volume (EDV) is the volume of blood in the ventricle at the end of diastole (filling phase).
- End-Systolic Volume (ESV) is the volume of blood remaining in the ventricle at the end of systole (contraction phase).

Factors Affecting Stroke Volume:

- Preload: The volume of blood in the ventricle at the end of diastole, which influences the stretch of cardiac muscle fibers and thus affects stroke volume.

- Afterload: The resistance against which the heart must pump blood, primarily determined by systemic vascular resistance.

- Contractility: The strength of the heart's contractions, which determines the amount of blood ejected with each beat.
- Heart Rate: Faster heart rates may decrease diastolic filling time, affecting stroke volume.

Clinical Significance:

Stroke volume is a critical parameter in assessing cardiac function and diagnosing various cardiovascular conditions, such as heart failure, valvular heart disease, and cardiomyopathies.

Changes in stroke volume can indicate alterations in cardiac output and hemodynamic stability, which are important considerations in managing critically ill patients, monitoring during surgery, and optimizing treatment in individuals with cardiovascular diseases.

Overall, stroke volume is a fundamental measure of cardiac performance, reflecting the heart's ability to pump blood efficiently and maintain adequate circulation throughout the body. Monitoring stroke volume provides valuable insights into cardiovascular function and guides clinical decision-making in various medical settings.

Peripheral resistance, also known as systemic vascular resistance (SVR) or total peripheral resistance (TPR), refers to the resistance encountered by blood flow in the systemic circulation. It represents the collective resistance offered by the blood vessels throughout the body, excluding those in the pulmonary circulation.

Here's how heart peripheral resistance factors into cardiovascular physiology:

- Vasculature: Peripheral resistance is primarily determined by the diameter of the blood vessels (arteries, arterioles, and capillaries) and their degree of constriction or dilation. Narrower vessels increase resistance, while wider vessels decrease it.

- Vascular Tone: The degree of constriction or dilation of blood vessels, known as vascular tone, is regulated by various factors, including the autonomic nervous system, hormones (such as adrenaline and noradrenaline), and local factors like metabolites and oxygen levels.

- Blood Pressure Regulation: Peripheral resistance plays a crucial role in regulating blood pressure. An increase in resistance, if not compensated by appropriate adjustments, can lead to elevated blood pressure (hypertension), whereas decreased resistance can result in low blood pressure (hypotension).

- Cardiac Afterload: Peripheral resistance directly influences the workload on the heart, known as afterload. Higher resistance increases the workload on the heart, requiring it to pump with greater force to overcome the resistance and maintain adequate blood flow to the tissues.

- Organ Perfusion: Peripheral resistance impacts blood flow distribution to different organs and tissues based on their metabolic demands. Changes in resistance can alter organ perfusion, affecting their function and overall systemic physiology.

- Clinical Implications: Abnormalities in peripheral resistance are associated with various cardiovascular conditions, including hypertension, atherosclerosis, and peripheral vascular disease. Modulating peripheral resistance is a key therapeutic target in managing these conditions and optimizing cardiovascular health.

Overall, peripheral resistance is a critical determinant of systemic vascular function and cardiovascular homeostasis. Understanding its regulation and clinical implications is essential for diagnosing and managing cardiovascular diseases and maintaining overall health.

The pulse wave coefficient (PWV) is a measure used in cardiovascular physiology to assess arterial stiffness, a key indicator of cardiovascular health. It measures the speed at which the pulse wave travels along the arterial tree, reflecting the elasticity and compliance of the arteries. Arterial stiffness is associated with aging, hypertension, atherosclerosis, and other cardiovascular diseases.

Here's how the pulse wave coefficient is calculated and its significance:

- Calculation: The pulse wave coefficient is typically calculated by measuring the time it takes for the pulse wave to travel between two arterial sites, usually the carotid and femoral arteries, and dividing the distance between these sites by the transit time. The formula is:

PWV = Distance between arterial sites (meters) / Transit time (seconds)

Measurement Techniques: Several techniques can be used to measure PWV, including:

- Arterial tonometry: Sensors are placed over the carotid and femoral arteries to detect pulse waveforms.

- Doppler ultrasound: Ultrasound probes are used to measure blood flow velocity in the carotid and femoral arteries.

- Pulse wave velocity devices: Specialized devices, such as tonometer or oscillometric cuffs, can directly measure PWV.

Significance:

Arterial stiffness and elevated PWV are independent predictors of cardiovascular risk and mortality. Higher PWV values indicate greater arterial stiffness and are associated with increased risk of adverse cardiovascular events, such as heart attacks and strokes.

PWV is considered a useful clinical tool for assessing cardiovascular health and risk stratification in individuals with hypertension, diabetes, and other cardiovascular risk factors.

Monitoring changes in PWV over time can help track the progression of arterial stiffness and assess the effectiveness of interventions aimed at improving cardiovascular health, such as lifestyle modifications and medications.

Clinical Applications:

PWV is used in clinical practice to identify individuals at higher risk of cardiovascular events and guide treatment decisions.

It may be incorporated into cardiovascular risk assessment algorithms to improve risk stratification and inform treatment strategies.

Research suggests that interventions aimed at reducing arterial stiffness and lowering PWV, such as antihypertensive medications, exercise, and dietary modifications, may help improve cardiovascular outcomes and reduce mortality.

In summary, the pulse wave coefficient (PWV) is a valuable measure of arterial stiffness and cardiovascular risk. By assessing PWV, healthcare providers can gain insights into vascular health and make informed decisions regarding prevention, diagnosis, and management of cardiovascular diseases.

Cerebrovascular blood oxygen saturation refers to the level of oxygen saturation in the blood vessels supplying the brain, specifically the cerebral arteries and arterioles. It is an important parameter in understanding cerebral oxygenation and perfusion, which are critical for brain function and overall neurological health.

Here's a breakdown of cerebrovascular blood oxygen saturation and its significance:

- Measurement: Cerebrovascular blood oxygen saturation can be measured using various techniques, including:

- Near-infrared spectroscopy (NIRS): This non-invasive technique uses light to measure oxygen saturation levels in cerebral tissue. It provides continuous monitoring and can detect changes in cerebral oxygenation in real time.
- Invasive techniques: In some clinical settings, such as during neurosurgery or critical care, invasive methods like intra-arterial blood gas sampling or jugular venous oxygen saturation monitoring may be used to assess cerebral oxygenation.

Significance:

Cerebrovascular blood oxygen saturation reflects the balance between oxygen supply and demand in the brain. Adequate oxygenation is essential for normal brain function and cognitive processes.

Changes in cerebrovascular blood oxygen saturation can occur in various neurological conditions, including stroke, traumatic brain injury, cerebral ischemia, and neurodegenerative diseases. Monitoring these changes can provide valuable insights into disease progression and guide treatment decisions.

Maintaining optimal cerebrovascular blood oxygen saturation is particularly important during critical care interventions, such as anesthesia, mechanical ventilation, and hemodynamic management, to prevent cerebral hypoxia and minimize the risk of neurological complications.

Clinical Applications:

Cerebrovascular blood oxygen saturation monitoring is used in various clinical settings, including neurosurgery, intensive care units, and neonatal care, to assess cerebral oxygenation and perfusion.

It is utilized in the management of conditions such as stroke, traumatic brain injury, intracranial hemorrhage, and cardiac arrest to guide treatment and optimize neurological outcomes.

Continuous monitoring of cerebrovascular blood oxygen saturation allows healthcare providers to detect changes in cerebral oxygenation early and intervene promptly to prevent neurological damage.

In summary, cerebrovascular blood oxygen saturation is a crucial parameter in assessing cerebral oxygenation and perfusion. Monitoring changes in cerebrovascular oxygen saturation can help identify neurological disorders, guide treatment strategies, and optimize outcomes in various clinical settings.

Cerebrovascular blood oxygen volume refers to the total amount of oxygen carried by the blood vessels supplying the brain. It is a measure of the oxygen content within the cerebral circulation and plays a critical role in maintaining brain function and overall neurological health.

However, it's important to clarify that the term "cerebrovascular blood oxygen volume" is not commonly used in medical literature or clinical practice. Instead, healthcare providers and researchers typically focus on parameters such as cerebral blood flow, cerebral oxygen saturation, and cerebral oxygen extraction fraction to assess cerebral oxygenation and perfusion.

Here are some related concepts that are commonly used to evaluate cerebral oxygenation:

- Cerebral Blood Flow (CBF): Cerebral blood flow refers to the volume of blood flowing through the cerebral circulation per unit of time (usually measured in milliliters per minute). Adequate CBF is essential for delivering oxygen and nutrients to brain tissue and removing metabolic waste products.

- Cerebral Oxygen Saturation: Cerebral oxygen saturation, also known as regional cerebral oxygen saturation (rSO2), measures the percentage of hemoglobin in the cerebral circulation that is saturated with oxygen. It provides information about the balance between oxygen supply and demand in the brain.

- Cerebral Oxygen Extraction Fraction (OEF): Cerebral oxygen extraction fraction is the ratio of oxygen extracted by the brain to the total oxygen content delivered by the blood. It reflects the efficiency of oxygen utilization by brain tissue and can be altered in conditions such as ischemia or hypoxia.

- Oxygen Delivery to the Brain: Oxygen delivery to the brain depends on factors such as arterial oxygen content, cerebral blood flow, and cerebral oxygen extraction. Monitoring these parameters allows healthcare providers to assess cerebral oxygenation and make informed decisions regarding patient care.

In clinical practice, various techniques, including near-infrared spectroscopy (NIRS), positron emission tomography (PET), magnetic resonance imaging (MRI), and invasive monitoring methods, may be used to assess cerebral oxygenation and perfusion. These tools help healthcare providers evaluate brain function, diagnose neurological conditions, and guide treatment strategies to optimize cerebral oxygenation and maintain neurological health.

Cerebral Oxygen Partial Pressure (PO_2): This refers to the partial pressure of oxygen dissolved in the blood within the cerebral circulation. Cerebral PO_2 is a critical indicator of oxygen availability to brain tissue and is influenced by factors such as arterial oxygen content, cerebral blood flow, and cerebral oxygen extraction fraction. Monitoring cerebral PO_2 can provide insights into the adequacy of oxygen delivery to the brain and help assess cerebral oxygenation status.

Cerebral Perfusion Pressure (CPP): Cerebral perfusion pressure represents the pressure gradient that drives blood flow to the brain. It is calculated as the difference between mean arterial pressure (MAP) and intracranial pressure (ICP):

CPP = MAP - ICP

Maintaining an adequate CPP is crucial for ensuring sufficient cerebral blood flow and oxygen delivery to meet the metabolic demands of brain tissue. Decreases in CPP can lead to cerebral ischemia and impaired neurological function.

In clinical practice, monitoring cerebral oxygenation and perfusion is essential for assessing brain health and managing various neurological conditions, including traumatic brain injury, stroke, and cerebral ischemia. Healthcare providers may use invasive techniques such as intracranial pressure monitoring and cerebral oxygen saturation monitoring, as well as non-invasive methods like near-infrared spectroscopy (NIRS), to evaluate cerebral oxygenation and perfusion parameters and guide treatment decisions.

BLOOD LIPIDS

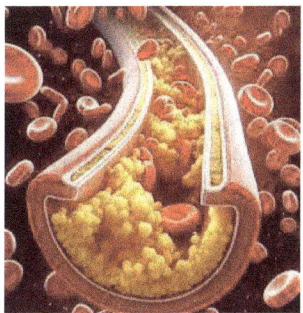

Blood viscosity refers to the thickness or resistance to flow of blood within the circulatory system. It is influenced by several factors, including the composition of blood, the presence of cells and proteins, and the shear forces exerted on the blood vessels. Blood viscosity plays a crucial role in cardiovascular health and can affect various aspects of circulatory function.

Here are some key points about blood viscosity:

- Composition of Blood: Blood is composed of plasma, red blood cells (erythrocytes), white blood cells (leukocytes), and platelets (thrombocytes). The viscosity of blood depends on the concentration and size of these components. Higher levels of red blood cells and proteins, such as fibrinogen, can increase blood viscosity.

- Hematocrit: Hematocrit refers to the proportion of red blood cells in the blood. An elevated hematocrit, indicating a higher concentration of red blood cells, can increase blood viscosity and impair circulation, leading to conditions such as thrombosis and hypertension.

- Shear Rate: Blood viscosity is not constant and can change depending on the shear rate, or the rate at which blood flows through the blood vessels. At higher shear rates, such as in arteries during exercise, blood viscosity decreases due to the deformation of red blood cells and the reduction in cell-

cell interactions. Conversely, at lower shear rates, such as in capillaries and veins, blood viscosity increases.

- Clinical Implications: Abnormalities in blood viscosity can have significant clinical implications. Increased blood viscosity is associated with conditions such as polycythemia, dehydration, hyperproteinemia, and hyperlipidemia, which can increase the risk of cardiovascular events such as heart attacks and strokes. Conversely, decreased blood viscosity may occur in conditions such as anemia and hypoproteinemia, leading to impaired oxygen delivery to tissues and organ dysfunction.

- Measurement: Blood viscosity can be measured directly using viscometers in laboratory settings. However, it is not routinely assessed in clinical practice. Instead, clinicians may indirectly evaluate blood viscosity by assessing hematocrit levels and other hematological parameters.

Overall, blood viscosity is an important determinant of circulatory function and cardiovascular health. Maintaining optimal blood viscosity is essential for ensuring efficient blood flow, oxygen delivery to tissues, and overall cardiovascular function.

Total cholesterol is a measurement of the total amount of cholesterol in your blood. It includes various types of cholesterol, including low-density lipoprotein (LDL) cholesterol, high-density lipoprotein (HDL) cholesterol, and very-low-density lipoprotein (VLDL) cholesterol. Cholesterol is a type of fat that is essential for building cell membranes, producing certain hormones, and synthesizing vitamin D. However, having high levels of total cholesterol, particularly LDL cholesterol (often referred to as "bad" cholesterol), can increase the risk of cardiovascular diseases such as heart attack and stroke.

Here are some key points about total cholesterol:

- Measurement: Total cholesterol is typically measured in milligrams per deciliter (mg/dL) of blood. A blood test called a lipid panel or lipid profile is used to measure total cholesterol along with other lipid components.

- Components: Total cholesterol includes several components:

LDL cholesterol: Often referred to as "bad" cholesterol because it can build up in the walls of your arteries and form plaque, which can narrow and block blood vessels.

HDL cholesterol: Often referred to as "good" cholesterol because it helps remove LDL cholesterol from the bloodstream and transport it to the liver for excretion.

VLDL cholesterol: Contains mostly triglycerides and is a precursor to LDL cholesterol. High levels of VLDL cholesterol are associated with an increased risk of cardiovascular disease.

Guidelines: According to guidelines from organizations such as the American Heart Association (AHA) and the National Heart, Lung, and Blood Institute (NHLBI), desirable levels of total cholesterol are as follows:

Total cholesterol: Less than 200 mg/dL is considered desirable.

LDL cholesterol: Less than 100 mg/dL is optimal for most people, although this target may vary based on individual risk factors.

HDL cholesterol: Higher levels are generally better, with levels above 60 mg/dL considered protective against heart disease.

- Risk Factors: Several factors can influence your total cholesterol levels, including genetics, diet, physical activity, age, gender, and certain medical conditions such as diabetes and hypothyroidism. High levels of total cholesterol, particularly LDL cholesterol, are considered a major risk factor for developing cardiovascular diseases.

- Management: Lifestyle changes, such as adopting a heart-healthy diet, increasing physical activity, maintaining a healthy weight, and quitting smoking, can help lower total cholesterol levels and reduce the risk of cardiovascular diseases. In some cases, medications such as statins may be prescribed to lower cholesterol levels further, particularly if lifestyle changes alone are not sufficient.

Overall, monitoring total cholesterol levels and managing other lipid components are essential for maintaining cardiovascular health and reducing the risk of heart disease and stroke. Regular screenings and discussions with your healthcare provider can help you understand your cholesterol levels and develop a personalized plan to improve your heart health.

Triglycerides are a type of fat (lipid) found in your blood. They are the most common type of fat in the body and are stored in fat cells for later use as energy. Triglycerides come from the foods you eat, especially from fats and carbohydrates.

Here are some key points about triglycerides:

- Measurement: Triglyceride levels are measured in milligrams per deciliter (mg/dL) of blood. Like total cholesterol, triglycerides are often measured as part of a lipid panel or lipid profile blood test.

- Role in the Body: Triglycerides serve as an energy source for the body. When you consume more calories than your body needs for immediate energy, the excess calories are converted into triglycerides and stored in fat cells. Between meals, hormones release triglycerides for energy between meals, hormones release triglycerides for energy.

- Relationship to Health: While triglycerides are necessary for good health, high levels of triglycerides in the blood can increase the risk of heart disease, particularly when combined with other risk factors such as high LDL cholesterol, low HDL cholesterol, and high blood pressure. High triglyceride levels are also associated with other health conditions, including obesity, metabolic syndrome, type 2 diabetes, and fatty liver disease.

Risk Factors: Several factors can contribute to high triglyceride levels, including:

- Diet high in saturated fats, trans fats, sugars, and refined carbohydrates
- Excess calorie intake and obesity
- Lack of physical activity
- Smoking
- Excessive alcohol consumption
- Certain medications, such as corticosteroids, estrogen, beta-blockers, and some diuretics

- Management: Lifestyle changes, such as adopting a heart-healthy diet low in saturated fats and sugars, increasing physical activity, losing weight if overweight or obese, quitting smoking, limiting alcohol intake, and managing underlying conditions such as diabetes and hypothyroidism, can help lower triglyceride levels. In some cases, medications such as statins, fibrates, niacin, and omega-3 fatty acids may be prescribed to lower triglyceride levels further.

Overall, maintaining healthy triglyceride levels is important for heart health and overall well-being. Regular screenings and discussions with your healthcare provider can help you understand your triglyceride levels and develop a personalized plan to improve your heart health.

High-density lipoprotein (HDL) is a type of lipoprotein, which is a complex of lipids (fats) and proteins that transports cholesterol and triglycerides through the bloodstream. HDL is often referred to as "good" cholesterol because it plays a crucial role in removing excess cholesterol from the bloodstream and transporting it to the liver for excretion, which helps protect against the development of atherosclerosis and cardiovascular disease.

Here are some key points about HDL cholesterol:

- Role in the Body: HDL cholesterol has several important functions:

- Reverse Cholesterol Transport: HDL picks up excess cholesterol from the walls of arteries and other tissues and transports it back to the liver for elimination from the body, a process known as reverse cholesterol transport.

- Antioxidant and Anti-inflammatory Effects: HDL has antioxidant and anti-inflammatory properties that help protect against damage to blood vessel walls and reduce inflammation, both of which are associated with the development of atherosclerosis and cardiovascular disease.

- Endothelial Function: HDL promotes the health and function of the endothelium, the inner lining of blood vessels, helping maintain vascular health and integrity.

- Measurement: HDL cholesterol levels are typically measured in milligrams per deciliter (mg/dL) of blood. A blood test called a lipid panel or lipid profile is used to measure HDL cholesterol along with other lipid components.

- Guidelines: According to guidelines from organizations such as the American Heart Association (AHA) and the National Heart, Lung, and Blood Institute (NHLBI), higher levels of HDL cholesterol are generally associated with a lower risk of cardiovascular disease. Desirable levels of HDL cholesterol are typically:

For men: Greater than 40 mg/dL

For women: Greater than 50 mg/dL Higher levels of HDL cholesterol are considered protective against heart disease, while lower levels are associated with an increased risk.

Factors Affecting HDL Levels: Several factors can influence HDL cholesterol levels, including:

- Genetics: HDL cholesterol levels can be influenced by genetic factors.

- Diet: Certain dietary factors, such as consuming healthy fats (such as those found in olive oil, fatty fish, nuts, and avocados), moderate alcohol consumption, and regular physical activity, can help raise HDL levels.

- Lifestyle: Factors such as smoking, obesity, sedentary lifestyle, and certain medical conditions (such as type 2 diabetes and metabolic syndrome) can lower HDL levels.

- Clinical Significance: Monitoring HDL cholesterol levels is important for assessing cardiovascular risk and guiding treatment decisions. Increasing HDL cholesterol levels through lifestyle modifications (such as diet and exercise) and, in some cases, medication (such as statins or fibrates) can help reduce the risk of cardiovascular disease.

Overall, HDL cholesterol plays a crucial role in cardiovascular health by helping to remove excess cholesterol from the bloodstream and protect against the development of atherosclerosis and cardiovascular disease. Maintaining optimal levels of HDL cholesterol through lifestyle modifications and, if necessary, medication can help promote heart health and reduce the risk of cardiovascular events.

Low-density lipoprotein (LDL) is a type of lipoprotein, a complex of lipids (fats) and proteins that transports cholesterol and triglycerides through the bloodstream. LDL is often referred to as "bad" cholesterol because high levels of LDL cholesterol are associated with an increased risk of atherosclerosis and cardiovascular disease.

Here are some key points about LDL cholesterol:

- Role in the Body: LDL cholesterol plays a critical role in delivering cholesterol to cells throughout the body. However, when LDL cholesterol levels are elevated, excess cholesterol can accumulate in the walls of arteries, leading to the formation of plaques. Over time, these plaques can narrow and block blood vessels, increasing the risk of heart attack, stroke, and other cardiovascular events.

- Measurement: LDL cholesterol levels are typically measured in milligrams per deciliter (mg/dL) of blood. A blood test called a lipid panel or lipid profile is used to measure LDL cholesterol along with other lipid components.

- Guidelines: According to guidelines from organizations such as the American Heart Association (AHA) and the National Heart, Lung, and Blood Institute (NHLBI), desirable levels of LDL cholesterol depend on an individual's cardiovascular risk factors:

For individuals with no other risk factors for heart disease, an LDL cholesterol level below 100 mg/dL is considered optimal.

For individuals with one or more risk factors for heart disease (such as smoking, high blood pressure, family history of heart disease, or diabetes), a lower LDL cholesterol level may be recommended (typically below 70-100 mg/dL, depending on individual risk factors).

Factors Affecting LDL Levels: Several factors can influence LDL cholesterol levels, including:

- Diet: Consuming a diet high in saturated and trans fats, cholesterol, and processed foods can increase LDL cholesterol levels.

- Genetics: Genetic factors can influence LDL cholesterol levels, with some individuals having a genetic predisposition to high LDL cholesterol levels.
- Lifestyle: Factors such as obesity, physical inactivity, smoking, and excessive alcohol consumption can contribute to elevated LDL cholesterol levels.

- Medical Conditions: Certain medical conditions, such as diabetes, hypothyroidism, and chronic kidney disease, can affect LDL cholesterol levels.

- Clinical Significance: Monitoring LDL cholesterol levels is important for assessing cardiovascular risk and guiding treatment decisions. Lifestyle modifications, such as adopting a heart-healthy diet, increasing physical activity, losing weight if overweight or obese, quitting smoking, and managing underlying medical conditions, can help lower LDL cholesterol levels. In some cases, medications such as statins or other cholesterol-lowering drugs may be prescribed to further reduce LDL cholesterol levels and reduce the risk of cardiovascular events.

Overall, maintaining optimal LDL cholesterol levels is essential for promoting heart health and reducing the risk of cardiovascular disease. Regular screenings and discussions with your healthcare provider can help you understand your LDL cholesterol levels and develop a personalized plan to improve your heart health.

Neutral fat" is a term that is often used interchangeably with "triglycerides" in the context of biochemistry and nutrition. Triglycerides are the most common type of fat found in the body and in the diet. They consist of a glycerol molecule attached to three fatty acid chains.

Here's a breakdown of neutral fat (triglycerides) and their significance:

- Chemical Structure: Triglycerides consist of three fatty acids attached to a glycerol molecule. The fatty acids can vary in length and degree of saturation, which affects the physical properties and metabolic fate of the triglycerides.

- Storage and Energy: Triglycerides are the main form of energy storage in the body. They are stored in adipose tissue (fat cells) and can be broken down into fatty acids and glycerol when the body needs energy. Triglycerides provide more than twice the energy per gram compared to carbohydrates and proteins, making them an efficient energy source.

- Dietary Sources: Triglycerides are found in various foods, particularly those high in fats and oils. Common dietary sources of triglycerides include fatty meats, dairy products, cooking oils, nuts, seeds, and processed foods containing added fats and oils.

- Metabolism: Triglycerides are broken down (hydrolyzed) by enzymes called lipases into fatty acids and glycerol, which are then absorbed into the bloodstream and transported to tissues for energy production. Excess triglycerides that are not immediately needed for energy are stored in adipose tissue.

- Health Implications: Elevated levels of triglycerides in the blood (hypertriglyceridemia) are associated with an increased risk of cardiovascular disease, particularly when combined with other risk factors such as high LDL cholesterol, low HDL cholesterol, and high blood pressure. Hypertriglyceridemia can be caused by various factors, including obesity, physical inactivity, excessive alcohol consumption, uncontrolled diabetes, and certain medications.

- Management: Lifestyle modifications, such as adopting a healthy diet low in saturated fats and sugars, increasing physical activity, losing weight if overweight or obese, quitting smoking, and limiting alcohol intake, can help lower triglyceride levels. In some cases, medications such as fibrates or omega-3 fatty acid supplements may be prescribed to lower triglyceride levels further.

Overall, triglycerides (neutral fat) play a crucial role in energy metabolism and are an important component of the diet. Maintaining optimal triglyceride levels through healthy lifestyle habits is essential for promoting heart health and reducing the risk of cardiovascular disease. Regular screenings and discussions with your healthcare provider can help you understand your triglyceride levels and develop a personalized plan to improve your overall health.

Circulating immune complexes (CICs) are soluble antigen-antibody complexes that are formed in the bloodstream when antibodies bind to antigens, such as pathogens or foreign substances. These complexes play a role in the body's immune response and can be detected in the blood during certain immune-mediated diseases and conditions.

Here's a breakdown of circulating immune complexes and their significance:

- Formation: Circulating immune complexes are formed when antibodies produced by the immune system bind to antigens, forming complexes that circulate in the bloodstream. Antigens can include foreign pathogens, such as bacteria, viruses, or fungi, as well as non-pathogenic substances, such as food antigens or environmental allergens.

- Role in Immune Response: Circulating immune complexes play a dual role in the immune response. On one hand, they can help neutralize and eliminate antigens by tagging them for removal by immune cells, such as macrophages and neutrophils. On the other hand, excessive formation of immune complexes or impaired clearance mechanisms can lead to inflammation and tissue damage, contributing to the pathogenesis of autoimmune diseases and immune-mediated disorders.

- Detection and Measurement: Circulating immune complexes can be detected and measured in the blood using various laboratory techniques, such as enzyme-linked immunosorbent assay (ELISA), immunodiffusion, or immunofluorescence assays. Quantitative measurement of CICs may be used as a diagnostic or prognostic marker for certain autoimmune diseases, infectious diseases, inflammatory conditions, and other immune-related disorders.

- Clinical Significance: Abnormal levels of circulating immune complexes have been associated with various diseases and conditions, including:
- Autoimmune diseases: Such as systemic lupus erythematous (SLE), rheumatoid arthritis, and autoimmune vasculitis.

- Infectious diseases: Such as viral infections (e.g., hepatitis B and C, HIV), bacterial infections (e.g., bacterial endocarditis), and parasitic infections (e.g., malaria).

- Inflammatory disorders: Such as immune complex-mediated glomerulonephritis, serum sickness, and hypersensitivity reactions.

- Cancer: Certain malignancies may lead to the production of circulating immune complexes, although their role in cancer pathogenesis is not fully understood.

- Treatment and Management: The management of conditions associated with circulating immune complexes depends on the underlying cause and may include treatment with immunosuppressive medications, anti-inflammatory agents, or targeted therapies directed at reducing immune complex formation or inflammation.

Overall, circulating immune complexes are an important component of the body's immune response and can serve as valuable biomarkers for diagnosing and monitoring immune-related diseases and conditions. Understanding the role of CICs in health and disease can help guide clinical management and improve patient outcomes.

PROSTATE

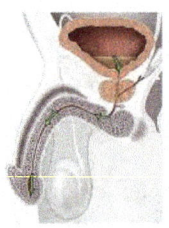 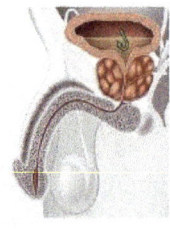

The degree of prostatic hyperplasia, also known as benign prostatic hyperplasia (BPH), refers to the extent or severity of enlargement of the prostate gland. BPH is a common condition where the prostate gland gradually enlarges as men age, often causing urinary symptoms due to compression of the urethra.

Clinically, the degree of prostatic hyperplasia is typically assessed through various methods, *including:*

- Digital Rectal Examination (DRE): During a DRE, a healthcare provider inserts a gloved, lubricated finger into the rectum to feel the size, shape, and consistency of the prostate gland. The degree of enlargement can be subjectively assessed based on this examination.

Imaging Studies: Imaging studies such as transrectal ultrasound (TRUS) or MRI can provide more detailed information about the size and morphology of the prostate gland, helping to assess the degree of hyperplasia.

- Symptom Severity: The severity of symptoms experienced by the patient, such as urinary frequency, urgency, weak urinary stream, incomplete emptying of the bladder, etc., can also provide an indication of the degree of prostatic hyperplasia.

- Uroflowmetry: Uroflowmetry is a test used to measure the flow rate of urine during urination. A reduced flow rate can be indicative of obstruction due to prostatic hyperplasia.

- Prostate-Specific Antigen (PSA) Level: While PSA levels are primarily used to screen for prostate cancer, they can also be elevated in men with BPH. However, PSA levels alone cannot determine the degree of hyperplasia.

Once the degree of prostatic hyperplasia is assessed, treatment options can be tailored accordingly. Mild cases may be managed conservatively with lifestyle modifications and medications, while more severe cases may require surgical intervention such as transurethral resection of the prostate (TURP) or laser surgery to alleviate symptoms and improve urinary flow.

The degree of prostatic calcification refers to the extent or severity of calcium deposits within the prostate gland. Prostatic calcifications are common and can be identified through imaging studies such as transrectal ultrasound (TRUS) or pelvic X-rays. The degree of prostatic calcification can vary from minimal to extensive.

Clinically, the degree of prostatic calcification is typically assessed based on the following characteristics:

- Size and Number: The size and number of calcifications within the prostate gland can vary. Small, isolated calcifications may be considered minimal, while larger or numerous calcifications may indicate a more extensive degree of calcification.

- Distribution: Prostatic calcifications can be distributed throughout the prostate gland or concentrated in specific areas. The distribution pattern may provide additional information about the degree of calcification and its potential impact on prostate health.

- Symptoms: In some cases, prostatic calcifications may be asymptomatic and incidentally discovered during imaging studies. However, extensive calcifications or calcifications located in specific areas of the prostate gland may contribute to urinary symptoms such as difficulty urinating, urinary frequency, or discomfort.

- Association with Other Conditions: Prostatic calcifications may be associated with certain conditions such as benign prostatic hyperplasia (BPH), chronic prostatitis, or prostate cancer. The presence of additional symptoms or findings may help clinicians assess the degree of calcification and its implications for overall prostate health.

Treatment for prostatic calcifications typically depends on the underlying cause and associated symptoms. In some cases, no treatment may be necessary if the calcifications are asymptomatic and not associated with underlying pathology. However, if prostatic calcifications contribute to urinary symptoms or are associated with other prostate conditions, treatment options may include medications, lifestyle modifications, or procedures to address underlying causes such as BPH or prostatitis. It's important for individuals with prostatic calcifications to consult with a healthcare professional for proper evaluation and management.

Prostatitis syndrome refers to a group of conditions characterized by inflammation or infection of the prostate gland. It's important to note that prostatitis syndrome encompasses a spectrum of conditions, ranging from acute bacterial prostatitis to chronic prostatitis/chronic pelvic pain syndrome (CP/CPPS). These conditions can cause a variety of symptoms and can have different causes and treatment approaches.

- Acute Bacterial Prostatitis: This is a sudden bacterial infection of the prostate gland. It can cause severe symptoms such as fever, chills, pain in the lower back and genital area, frequent and urgent urination, and difficulty urinating. Acute bacterial prostatitis is typically treated with antibiotics.

- Chronic Bacterial Prostatitis: This condition involves recurrent or persistent bacterial infections of the prostate gland. Symptoms may be less severe than acute bacterial prostatitis but can still include pelvic pain, urinary symptoms, and discomfort during ejaculation. Treatment usually involves long-term antibiotics.

- Chronic Prostatitis/Chronic Pelvic Pain Syndrome (CP/CPPS): This is the most common form of prostatitis and is characterized by pelvic pain and discomfort lasting at least three months without evidence of bacterial infection. It can also involve urinary symptoms, sexual dysfunction, and psychological distress. The exact cause of CP/CPPS is often unclear, and treatment may involve a combination of medications (such as alpha-blockers, anti-inflammatory drugs, or muscle relaxants), physical therapy, lifestyle changes, and psychological support.

- Asymptomatic Inflammatory Prostatitis: Some men may have inflammation of the prostate gland without experiencing any symptoms. This condition is often diagnosed incidentally during evaluation for other prostate-related issues or through tests such as prostate-specific antigen (PSA) screening.

Prostatitis syndrome can significantly impact quality of life and may require a multidisciplinary approach to management, involving urologists, primary care physicians, pain specialists, and other healthcare providers. Treatment is often tailored to the specific type and severity of prostatitis, as well as individual patient factors. It's essential for individuals experiencing symptoms suggestive of prostatitis to seek medical evaluation for proper diagnosis and management.

MALE SEXUAL FUNCTION

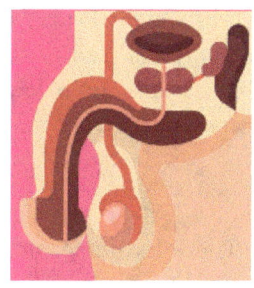

A hormone primarily produced in the testicles in men and in smaller amounts in the ovaries and adrenal glands in women. Testosterone plays a crucial role in various physiological processes, *including:*

- Development of Male Reproductive Tissues: Testosterone is responsible for the development and maintenance of male reproductive tissues, including the testes and prostate gland.

- Sexual Function: Testosterone influences libido (sex drive) and is essential for the development of male secondary sexual characteristics such as facial and body hair, deepening of the voice, and muscle mass.

- Bone Density: Testosterone contributes to bone density and strength, helping to prevent osteoporosis and maintain overall bone health.
- Muscle Mass and Strength: Testosterone promotes the growth and maintenance of lean muscle mass and helps regulate muscle strength and function.

- Fat Distribution: Testosterone influences fat distribution in the body, with lower levels associated with increased fat mass, particularly around the abdomen.

- Mood and Cognitive Function: Testosterone levels can affect mood, cognitive function, and overall sense of well-being. Low testosterone levels have been associated with symptoms such as fatigue, depression, and decreased cognitive function.

Testosterone levels naturally decline with age, typically starting in the late 20s or early 30s, at a rate of about 1% per year. In some cases, low testosterone levels (also known as hypogonadism) can occur due to certain medical conditions, medications, or lifestyle factors. Symptoms of low testosterone may include decreased libido, erectile dysfunction, fatigue, reduced muscle mass, and mood changes.

Treatment for low testosterone may involve hormone replacement therapy (such as testosterone replacement therapy), lifestyle modifications (such as weight loss and exercise), and management of underlying medical conditions contributing to low testosterone levels. It's important for individuals experiencing symptoms of low testosterone to consult with a healthcare professional for proper evaluation and management.

Gonadotropins are a type of hormone that act on the gonads, which are the reproductive organs (ovaries in females and testes in males). These hormones are produced by the anterior pituitary gland, a small gland located at the base of the brain. Gonadotropins play a crucial role in regulating the growth, development, and function of the gonads, as well as the production of sex hormones.

There are two primary gonadotropins:

- Follicle-stimulating hormone (FSH): In females, FSH stimulates the growth and development of ovarian follicles (small sacs within the ovaries that contain eggs) during the menstrual cycle. It also triggers the production of estrogen by the ovarian follicles. In males, FSH stimulates the production of sperm (spermatogenesis) in the testes.

- Luteinizing hormone (LH): In females, LH works in conjunction with FSH to regulate the menstrual cycle and ovulation. It stimulates the release of a mature egg from the ovary (ovulation) and promotes the production of progesterone by the corpus luteum (a structure formed after ovulation). In males, LH stimulates the production of testosterone by the Leydig cells in the testes.

The secretion of gonadotropins is controlled by the hypothalamus-pituitary-gonadal (HPG) axis, a complex feedback system involving interactions between the hypothalamus, pituitary gland, and gonads. Gonadotropin-releasing hormone (GnRH), produced by the hypothalamus, stimulates the release of FSH and LH from the anterior pituitary gland. In turn, FSH and LH regulate the production of sex hormones (estrogen and progesterone in females, testosterone in males) and gamete development (oogenesis and spermatogenesis).

Disorders of gonadotropin production or function can lead to various reproductive health issues, including infertility, menstrual irregularities, and disorders of sexual development. In assisted reproductive technologies (ART), synthetic forms of gonadotropins are often used to stimulate follicle development in women undergoing ovulation induction for fertility treatment.

Overall, gonadotropins play a crucial role in the regulation of reproductive function and fertility in both males and females.

The process of achieving and maintaining an erection. Neurotransmitters are chemical messengers that transmit signals between nerve cells (neurons) and play a crucial role in various physiological processes, including sexual arousal and erectile function.

Several neurotransmitters are involved in the complex process of penile erection. These include:

- Nitric oxide (NO): Nitric oxide is a key neurotransmitter involved in the relaxation of smooth muscle cells in the blood vessels of the penis. It is produced by endothelial cells lining the blood vessels and acts to dilate blood vessels, allowing increased blood flow into the penis, which is essential for achieving and maintaining an erection. Medications such as sildenafil (Viagra), tadalafil (Cialis), and vardenafil (Levitra) work by enhancing the effects of nitric oxide.

- Acetylcholine: Acetylcholine is another neurotransmitter involved in penile erection. It acts on nerve endings in the penis to stimulate the release of nitric oxide and promote smooth muscle relaxation, leading to increased blood flow into the erectile tissues.

- Dopamine: Dopamine is a neurotransmitter associated with feelings of pleasure and reward. It plays a role in the brain's response to sexual stimuli and can enhance sexual arousal. Dysfunction in the dopaminergic system has been implicated in certain types of erectile dysfunction.

- Serotonin: Serotonin is a neurotransmitter that plays a role in mood regulation and emotional states. It can have both excitatory and inhibitory effects on sexual function, depending on the context. Imbalances in serotonin levels may contribute to sexual dysfunction, including erectile dysfunction.
- Norepinephrine: Norepinephrine is involved in the sympathetic nervous system's response to stress and arousal. In the context of sexual function, it can have both excitatory and inhibitory effects, depending on the balance between sympathetic and parasympathetic activity.

- Oxytocin: Oxytocin is often referred to as the "love hormone" and is associated with social bonding and attachment. It may play a role in sexual arousal and intimacy, although its specific effects on erectile function are not fully understood.

Overall, the interplay of neurotransmitters within the central and peripheral nervous systems is crucial for the regulation of erectile function. Dysfunction in any of these neurotransmitter systems can contribute to erectile dysfunction, a common condition characterized by the inability to achieve or maintain an erection sufficient for satisfactory sexual performance.

Semen volume refers to the amount of fluid ejaculated during ejaculation. Semen is composed of various components, including spermatozoa (sperm cells) and seminal fluid, which is produced by accessory reproductive glands such as the seminal vesicles, prostate gland, and bulbourethral glands. *The volume of semen can vary among individuals and can be influenced by various factors, including:*

- Frequency of Ejaculation: The frequency of ejaculation can affect semen volume. Generally, longer periods of abstinence may lead to a larger volume of semen upon ejaculation, whereas more frequent ejaculation may result in smaller volumes.

- Hydration Status: Adequate hydration is important for maintaining normal semen volume. Dehydration can lead to decreased semen volume and concentration.
- Age: Semen volume typically peaks in young adulthood and may gradually decrease with age. However, this decline is often subtle and may not significantly affect fertility.

- Sexual Arousal: The level of sexual arousal can influence semen volume. Higher levels of arousal may lead to larger volumes of ejaculate.

- Health and Lifestyle Factors: Certain health and lifestyle factors can impact semen volume. For example, smoking, excessive alcohol consumption, obesity, and poor diet can negatively affect semen quality and volume. Conversely, regular exercise, a balanced diet, and avoidance of harmful substances may help maintain healthy semen parameters.

- Medical Conditions and Medications: Certain medical conditions, such as hormonal imbalances, genital infections, and prostate disorders, can affect semen volume. Additionally, some medications may have side effects that impact semen production.

While semen volume is one aspect of male fertility, it's important to note that fertility also depends on other factors, including sperm count, sperm motility (ability to swim), and sperm morphology (shape and size). If you have concerns about semen volume or fertility, it's advisable to consult with a healthcare provider or reproductive specialist for evaluation and guidance. They can perform appropriate tests to assess semen parameters and provide personalized recommendations based on your individual circumstances.

Liquefaction time refers to the duration it takes for semen to change from a gel-like consistency to a more liquid state after ejaculation. Normally, semen is ejaculated as a thick, gelatinous fluid, which is important for sperm to remain in the female reproductive tract following intercourse. Liquefaction is a natural process that enables sperm to swim freely and facilitates their journey through the female reproductive system.

The World Health Organization (WHO) guidelines suggest that normal liquefaction time for semen is typically within 20 to 30 minutes after ejaculation at body temperature (37°C or 98.6°F). During this time, enzymes from the prostate gland and seminal vesicles work to break down the gel-like consistency of the ejaculate, resulting in a more fluid consistency.

Abnormal liquefaction time prolonged or absent, can be indicative of certain underlying issues or conditions. Factors that may affect liquefaction time *include:*

- Infections: Infections of the male reproductive system, such as prostatitis or seminal vesiculitis, can interfere with the normal liquefaction process.

- Hormonal Imbalances: Hormonal imbalances, particularly involving testosterone or other reproductive hormones, may affect semen quality, including liquefaction time.

- Obstructions: Blockages or obstructions in the male reproductive tract can impede the flow of semen and affect liquefaction.

- Medications: Certain medications or medical treatments may impact semen liquefaction time as a side effect.

- Age: Aging may affect the composition and function of seminal fluid, potentially influencing liquefaction time.

If there are concerns about semen liquefaction time or fertility, it's advisable to consult with a healthcare provider or fertility specialist. They can perform a comprehensive evaluation, including semen analysis, to assess various parameters of semen quality and determine if any underlying issues need to be addressed.

The number of sperm cells present in a semen sample is typically measured as part of a semen analysis, which is a standard diagnostic test used to evaluate male fertility. Sperm count, or sperm concentration, refers to the concentration of sperm cells in a given volume of semen.

The World Health Organization (WHO) provides reference values for sperm parameters, including sperm count. According to the WHO guidelines, a normal sperm count is typically considered to be at least 15 million sperm per milliliter (mL) of semen. However, it's important to note that fertility can still be achieved with lower sperm counts, as fertility is influenced by various factors beyond just sperm count alone.

In addition to sperm count, other parameters assessed during a semen analysis include sperm motility (the percentage of sperm that are moving), sperm morphology (the percentage of sperm with a normal shape), semen volume, pH, and liquefaction time, among others. These parameters collectively provide valuable information about male fertility potential.

If there are concerns about sperm count or male fertility, it's recommended to consult with a healthcare provider or fertility specialist. They can perform a thorough evaluation, including a semen analysis, to assess sperm parameters and provide personalized recommendations based on individual circumstances. Additionally, they may investigate potential underlying causes of any abnormalities detected during testing.

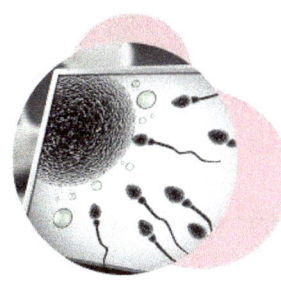

Sperm motility rate refers to the percentage of sperm cells in a semen sample that exhibit forward movement or progressive motility. Sperm motility is a crucial factor in male fertility because it determines the sperm's ability to swim through the female reproductive tract and fertilize an egg.

During a semen analysis, sperm motility is typically assessed by examining a sample of semen under a microscope. *Sperm cells are categorized into different motility categories based on their movement:*

- Progressive Motility: Sperm cells that move actively in a straight line or with large, sweeping motions.

- Non-Progressive Motility: Sperm cells that move, but their movement is not considered forward or directional.

- Immotile: Sperm cells that show no movement.

The total motility rate is the combined percentage of sperm cells exhibiting progressive and non-progressive motility.

The World Health Organization (WHO) provides reference values for sperm parameters, including sperm motility. According to the WHO guidelines, a normal total motility rate is typically considered to be at least 40% or higher. However, it's important to note that fertility can still be achieved with lower motility rates, as other factors such as sperm count and morphology also play a role.

Assessing sperm motility rate as part of a semen analysis provides valuable information about male fertility potential. If there are concerns about sperm motility or male fertility, it's recommended to consult with a healthcare provider or fertility specialist. They can perform a thorough evaluation, including a semen analysis, to assess sperm parameters and provide personalized recommendations based on individual circumstances. Additionally, they may investigate potential underlying causes of any abnormalities detected during testing.

GYNECOLOGY

Female hormones, also known as sex hormones, play crucial roles in the development, regulation, and maintenance of female reproductive functions and overall health. *The primary female hormones include*:

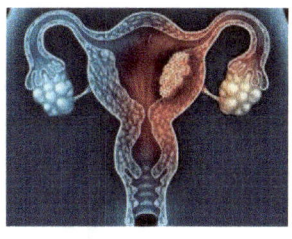

- Estrogens: Estrogens are a group of hormones responsible for the development and regulation of the female reproductive system. The three main types of estrogens in women are estradiol, estrone, and estriol. Estrogens are produced primarily by the ovaries, although small amounts are also produced by the adrenal glands and fat cells. Estrogens are involved in the development of secondary sexual characteristics, regulation of the menstrual cycle, maintenance of bone density, and modulation of mood and cognitive function.

- Progesterone: Progesterone is a hormone that works alongside estrogen to regulate the menstrual cycle and support pregnancy. It is primarily produced by the ovaries following ovulation. Progesterone helps prepare the uterus for implantation of a fertilized egg and supports early pregnancy by maintaining the uterine lining. If pregnancy does not occur, progesterone levels decrease, leading to menstruation.

- Follicle-Stimulating Hormone (FSH): FSH is produced by the anterior pituitary gland and plays a key role in the menstrual cycle and reproductive function. In women, FSH stimulates the growth and maturation of ovarian follicles (structures that contain developing eggs) during the follicular phase of the menstrual cycle.

- Luteinizing Hormone (LH): LH is also produced by the anterior pituitary gland and plays a crucial role in the menstrual cycle. In women, a surge in LH triggers ovulation, the release of a mature egg from the ovary. After ovulation, LH stimulates the development of the corpus luteum, a temporary endocrine gland that produces progesterone to support pregnancy.

These hormones work together in a tightly regulated feedback system known as the hypothalamic-pituitary-ovarian (HPO) axis to control the menstrual cycle and maintain reproductive function. Imbalances or disruptions in female hormone levels can lead to various reproductive health issues, including irregular menstrual cycles, infertility, polycystic ovary syndrome (PCOS), and menopausal symptoms.

It's important to note that hormone levels fluctuate throughout the menstrual cycle and change during different stages of a woman's life, such as puberty, pregnancy, and menopause. If you have concerns about your hormone levels or reproductive health, it's recommended to consult with a healthcare provider or gynecologist for evaluation and management.

Gonadotropins are a group of hormones that act on the gonads, which are the reproductive organs (testes in males and ovaries in females). These hormones are produced and secreted by the anterior pituitary gland, a pea-sized gland located at the base of the brain. Gonadotropins play crucial roles in regulating the growth, development, and function of the gonads, as well as the production of sex hormones.

There are two primary gonadotropins:

- Follicle-Stimulating Hormone (FSH): FSH plays a key role in the regulation of the reproductive system in both males and females. In females, FSH stimulates the growth and development of ovarian follicles (structures that contain developing eggs) during the follicular phase of the menstrual cycle. In males, FSH stimulates spermatogenesis, the process of sperm cell production in the testes.

- Luteinizing Hormone (LH): LH is involved in the regulation of the menstrual cycle and ovulation in females, as well as the production of sex hormones in both males and females. In females, a surge in LH triggers ovulation, the release of a mature egg from the ovary. After ovulation, LH stimulates the development of the corpus luteum, a temporary endocrine gland that produces progesterone to support pregnancy. In males, LH stimulates the Leydig cells in the testes to produce testosterone, the primary male sex hormone.

The secretion of gonadotropins is regulated by the hypothalamic-pituitary-gonadal (HPG) axis, a complex feedback system involving interactions between the hypothalamus, pituitary gland, and gonads. Gonadotropin-releasing hormone (GnRH), produced by the hypothalamus, stimulates the release of FSH and LH from the anterior pituitary gland. In turn, FSH and LH regulate the production of sex hormones (such as estrogen and progesterone in females, testosterone in males) and gamete development (oogenesis and spermatogenesis).

Disorders of gonadotropin production or function can lead to various reproductive health issues, including infertility, menstrual irregularities, and disorders of sexual development. In assisted reproductive technologies (ART), synthetic forms of gonadotropins are often used to stimulate follicle development in women undergoing ovulation induction for fertility treatment.

Overall, gonadotropins play crucial roles in the regulation of reproductive function and fertility in both males and females.

Prolactin is a peptide hormone produced and secreted by the anterior pituitary gland, a small gland located at the base of the brain. It plays a crucial role in various physiological processes, primarily related to reproduction and lactation in mammals. *Prolactin is involved in the following functions:*

- Stimulation of Milk Production: Prolactin is best known for its role in lactation. In females, especially during pregnancy and after childbirth, prolactin levels increase significantly to stimulate the development of mammary glands and milk production (lactogenesis). Prolactin continues to promote milk production as long as breastfeeding continues, and its levels are regulated by a feedback mechanism involving suckling and the release of another hormone, oxytocin.

- Regulation of Reproductive Function: Prolactin also plays a role in regulating reproductive function, although its exact mechanisms are complex and not fully understood. In females, high levels of prolactin can suppress ovulation (the release of eggs from the ovaries) and disrupt menstrual cycles, leading to infertility or irregular periods. In males, prolactin may influence testosterone production and sperm production, although its effects on male fertility are less clear.

- Immune Modulation: Prolactin has immunomodulatory effects and is involved in regulating the immune system's function. It plays a role in the development and function of immune cells and can influence immune responses to infection, inflammation, and autoimmune diseases.

- Behavioral Effects: Prolactin has been implicated in various behavioral and physiological responses, including maternal behavior, stress responses, and sexual behavior. However, its exact role in these processes is still being studied.

Abnormalities in prolactin levels can occur due to various factors, including medical conditions, medications, stress, and lifestyle factors. Hyperprolactinemia, or elevated levels of prolactin in the blood, can lead to symptoms such as irregular menstrual periods, infertility, galactorrhea (inappropriate milk production), and decreased libido. Hypoprolactinemia, or low levels of prolactin, may be associated with certain medical conditions but is less common.

If there are concerns about prolactin levels or associated symptoms, it's important to consult with a healthcare provider or endocrinologist for evaluation and management. Testing prolactin levels through blood tests can help diagnose hyperprolactinemia or other related conditions, and treatment options may include medications or addressing underlying causes.

Progesterone is a steroid hormone primarily produced by the ovaries in women, specifically by the corpus luteum following ovulation. It is also produced in smaller amounts by the adrenal glands. Progesterone plays crucial roles in the menstrual cycle, pregnancy, and various other physiological processes. Some key functions of progesterone *include:*

- Regulation of the Menstrual Cycle: Progesterone is involved in the regulation of the menstrual cycle, particularly during the luteal phase (the second half) of the cycle. After ovulation, progesterone levels rise, preparing the uterine lining (endometrium) for possible implantation of a fertilized egg. If pregnancy does not occur, progesterone levels decline, leading to menstruation.

- Support of Pregnancy: Progesterone is essential for the maintenance of pregnancy. After fertilization, progesterone helps maintain the uterine lining, ensuring a suitable environment for the developing embryo. Progesterone also helps prevent uterine contractions that could lead to premature labor and supports the development of the placenta, which provides oxygen and nutrients to the growing fetus.

- Development of Breast Tissue: Progesterone, along with estrogen, promotes the development of breast tissue and prepares the breasts for lactation during pregnancy.

- Regulation of Mood and Sleep: Progesterone has effects on the central nervous system and can influence mood, cognition, and sleep patterns. Changes in progesterone levels throughout the menstrual cycle may contribute to mood fluctuations and changes in sleep quality.
- Modulation of Immune Function: Progesterone has immunomodulatory effects and can influence the function of the immune system. It plays a role in maintaining immune tolerance during pregnancy, preventing the maternal immune system from rejecting the developing fetus.

- Other Functions: Progesterone also has effects on various other organs and tissues in the body, including the skin, bone, and cardiovascular system. It may also play a role in metabolic regulation and thermoregulation.

Progesterone levels fluctuate throughout the menstrual cycle, peaking during the luteal phase and declining before menstruation. In addition to its physiological roles, progesterone is also used therapeutically for various purposes, including hormone replacement therapy, fertility treatments, and the prevention of miscarriage in certain cases.

If there are concerns about progesterone levels or related symptoms, it's important to consult with a healthcare provider or gynecologist for evaluation and management. They can perform appropriate tests to assess progesterone levels and provide personalized recommendations based on individual circumstances.

Vaginitis" refers to inflammation of the vagina, which can result from various causes, including infections, hormonal changes, allergies, or irritants. *The most common types of vaginitis include*:

- Bacterial Vaginitis (BV): BV is caused by an imbalance of the bacteria normally found in the vagina. It often presents with a thin, white or gray vaginal discharge with a fishy odor.

- Yeast Infection (Candidiasis): Yeast infections are caused by an overgrowth of the fungus Candida albicans. Symptoms may include a thick, white, cottage cheese-like vaginal discharge, itching, and irritation.
- Trichomoniasis: Trichomoniasis is a sexually transmitted infection caused by the parasite Trichomonas vaginitis. It can cause vaginal itching, burning, redness, and a frothy, yellow-green vaginal discharge.

- Atrophic Vaginitis: Atrophic vaginitis occurs due to a decrease in estrogen levels, commonly seen in menopausal women. It may cause vaginal dryness, itching, burning, and discomfort during intercourse.

The term "coefficient" typically refers to a numerical or quantitative measure of a particular phenomenon. In the context of vaginitis, there are no coefficients commonly used to quantify the condition. Diagnosis and management of vaginitis usually involve clinical evaluation, medical history, physical examination, and sometimes laboratory tests (such as vaginal swabs or cultures) to identify the underlying cause.

Treatment for vaginitis depends on the specific cause and may include antifungal medications, antibiotics, or hormone therapy, as appropriate. It's essential for individuals experiencing symptoms of vaginitis to seek medical attention from a healthcare provider for proper diagnosis and management.

PID stands for Pelvic Inflammatory Disease, which is a serious infection of the female reproductive organs. It typically occurs when sexually transmitted bacteria spread from the vagina to the uterus, fallopian tubes, or ovaries.

Pelvic Inflammatory Disease (PID) can lead to various complications such as chronic pelvic pain, ectopic pregnancy, infertility, and an increased risk of ectopic pregnancy. PID is often caused by sexually transmitted infections (STIs) such as chlamydia and gonorrhea, although other bacteria can also be involved.

Diagnosis of PID is typically based on a combination of symptoms, pelvic examination findings, and sometimes laboratory tests such as urine tests, cervical cultures, or imaging studies like ultrasound or MRI.

Treatment for PID usually involves antibiotics to treat the underlying infection. In severe cases, hospitalization and intravenous antibiotics may be necessary. Prompt treatment is crucial to prevent complications and long-term damage to the reproductive organs.

If you're referring to a "PID coefficient" in a specific context, please provide more information, and I'd be happy to assist you further.

"Appendagitis" typically refers to inflammation of the appendages of the uterus, also known as the uterine appendages or adnexa. The adnexa include the fallopian tubes, ovaries, and supporting ligaments.

Inflammation of the uterine appendages can occur due to various reasons, including infections, torsion (twisting), or other inflammatory conditions. However, "appendagitis" is not a commonly used term in medical literature. It's possible that you may be referring to a specific condition or context related to inflammation or pathology of the uterine appendages.

If you have a specific question or concern related to appendagitis or inflammation of the uterine appendages, I would recommend providing additional context or details so that I can offer more relevant information. Alternatively, consulting with a healthcare provider or gynecologist would be advisable for proper evaluation and management. They can perform a thorough examination, order appropriate tests if needed, and provide personalized recommendations based on individual circumstances.

"Cervicitis" refers to inflammation of the cervix, which is the lower part of the uterus that connects to the vagina. This inflammation can be caused by various factors, including infections (such as sexually transmitted infections like chlamydia, gonorrhea, or genital herpes), irritation (such as from douching or using certain hygiene products), or allergic reactions.

There is no specific "cervicitis coefficient" in medical terminology. However, "coefficient" typically refers to a numerical value or factor used in a mathematical equation or statistical analysis. In the context of cervicitis, there may not be a single coefficient used to quantify the condition. Instead, diagnosis and management are typically based on clinical evaluation, medical history, physical examination findings (including cervical appearance and tenderness), and sometimes laboratory tests (such as cervical swabs or cultures) to identify the underlying cause of inflammation.

Treatment for cervicitis depends on the underlying cause. It may involve antibiotics for bacterial infections, antiviral medications for viral infections, or other treatments as appropriate. Avoiding irritants and practicing safe sex can help prevent cervicitis.

If you have concerns about cervicitis or are experiencing symptoms such as abnormal vaginal discharge, pelvic pain, or bleeding, it's important to consult with a healthcare provider or gynecologist for evaluation and management. They can perform necessary tests, provide a proper diagnosis, and recommend appropriate treatment based on your individual circumstances.

Ovarian cysts are fluid-filled sacs that develop on the ovaries. They are common and often harmless, resolving on their own without treatment. However, in some cases, ovarian cysts can cause symptoms or complications and may require medical intervention.

When discussing ovarian cysts, healthcare providers may consider various factors, measurements, or characteristics to assess their size, type, and potential impact. These may include:

- Size: Ovarian cysts can vary in size, ranging from small cysts that are only a few millimeters to larger cysts that are several centimeters in diameter. The size of a cyst can influence its management and potential for complications.

- Type: Ovarian cysts can be classified into different types based on their appearance, composition, and origin. Common types include functional cysts (such as follicular cysts and corpus luteum cysts), dermoid cysts (containing tissue like hair, skin, or teeth), endometriomas (related to endometriosis), and cystadenomas (developing from ovarian tissue).

- Symptoms: The presence of symptoms such as pelvic pain, bloating, pressure, or changes in menstrual cycles may indicate the presence of an ovarian cyst and may prompt further evaluation and management.

- Complications: Some ovarian cysts can lead to complications such as rupture, torsion (twisting), or hemorrhage. Assessing the risk of complications is important in determining the appropriate management approach.

- Imaging Findings: Imaging studies such as ultrasound or MRI can provide detailed information about the size, location, and characteristics of ovarian cysts, helping guide diagnosis and management decisions.

If you have concerns about ovarian cysts or are experiencing symptoms suggestive of their presence, it's important to consult with a healthcare provider or gynecologist for evaluation and management. They can perform necessary tests, provide a proper diagnosis, and recommend appropriate treatment based on your individual circumstances.

BREAST

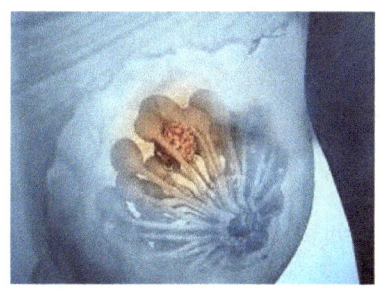

"**Hyperplasia of mammary glands**" refers to an increase in the number of cells within the breast tissue. This condition is commonly known as mammary gland hyperplasia or breast hyperplasia. It can occur due to various factors, including hormonal changes, medications, or underlying medical conditions. Mammary gland hyperplasia can present as breast enlargement, tenderness, or nodularity.

The term "coefficient" typically refers to a numerical factor or measure used in mathematical equations or statistical analysis.

If you have concerns about mammary gland hyperplasia or are experiencing symptoms such as breast enlargement or tenderness, it's important to consult with a healthcare provider or a breast specialist for evaluation and management. They can perform a clinical examination, order appropriate tests (such as imaging studies or biopsies if necessary), and recommend treatment options based on your individual circumstances. Treatment for mammary gland hyperplasia depends on the underlying cause and may include medications, hormonal therapy, or surgical intervention in some cases.

"Acute mastitis" refers to inflammation of the breast tissue, typically due to bacterial infection. It most commonly occurs in breastfeeding women, although it can also affect non-breastfeeding individuals. Acute mastitis often presents with symptoms such as breast pain, redness, warmth, swelling, and sometimes fever or chills.

There is no specific "coefficient" associated with acute mastitis in medical terminology. The term "coefficient" typically refers to a numerical factor or measure used in mathematical equations or statistical analysis. In the context of acute mastitis, clinical assessment, medical history, physical examination findings, and sometimes laboratory tests (such as breast milk culture) are used to diagnose the condition and guide treatment.

Treatment for acute mastitis usually involves a combination of antibiotics to treat the underlying bacterial infection and measures to relieve symptoms, such as pain management and warm compresses. It's important for individuals experiencing symptoms of acute mastitis to seek medical attention from a healthcare provider for proper evaluation and management. In severe cases or if complications develop (such as breast abscess formation), further interventions may be necessary, including drainage of the abscess.

If you have concerns about acute mastitis or are experiencing symptoms suggestive of the condition, it's important to consult with a healthcare provider for evaluation and appropriate management.

"Chronic mastitis" refers to long-standing inflammation of the breast tissue, which may persist over an extended period. It differs from acute mastitis, which is typically characterized by sudden onset and resolves with treatment. Chronic mastitis can present with symptoms such as breast pain, tenderness, swelling, and occasionally nipple discharge.

Similar to acute mastitis, there is no specific "coefficient" associated with chronic mastitis in medical terminology. The term "coefficient" typically refers to a numerical factor or measure used in mathematical equations or statistical analysis. In the context of chronic mastitis, diagnosis and management rely on clinical evaluation, medical history, physical examination findings, and sometimes imaging studies (such as ultrasound or MRI) and biopsy to assess the extent and nature of the inflammation.

Treatment for chronic mastitis depends on the underlying cause and may involve a combination of antibiotics (if bacterial infection is present), anti-inflammatory medications, warm compresses, supportive measures (such as wearing a well-fitted bra), and lifestyle modifications. In some cases, surgery may be necessary to remove affected breast tissue or abscesses.

If you have concerns about chronic mastitis or are experiencing symptoms suggestive of the condition, it's important to consult with a healthcare provider or breast specialist for evaluation and appropriate management. They can perform necessary tests, provide a proper diagnosis, and recommend treatment options based on your individual circumstances.

"**Endocrine dyscrasia**" refers to a disorder or imbalance involving the endocrine system, which is a network of glands that produce and secrete hormones to regulate various bodily functions. These glands include the pituitary, thyroid, parathyroid, adrenal, pancreas, ovaries, and testes. Hormones produced by these glands help regulate metabolism, growth and development, sexual function, mood, and other physiological processes.

In the context of endocrine dyscrasia, diagnosis and management depend on the specific hormonal imbalance or disorder present. Various endocrine disorders can cause dyscrasias, *including:*

- Hypothyroidism: Decreased thyroid hormone production by the thyroid gland.

- Hyperthyroidism: Excessive thyroid hormone production by the thyroid gland.

- Diabetes mellitus: Impaired insulin production or function, leading to abnormal blood sugar levels.

- Adrenal insufficiency: Inadequate production of adrenal hormones by the adrenal glands.

- Cushing's syndrome: Excessive cortisol production by the adrenal glands.

- Hypopituitarism: Reduced hormone production by the pituitary gland.
- Hyperparathyroidism: Overactivity of the parathyroid glands, leading to increased calcium levels in the blood.

Treatment for endocrine dyscrasia varies depending on the underlying cause and may include hormone replacement therapy, medications to regulate hormone levels, lifestyle modifications, and sometimes surgery. Management often requires collaboration between endocrinologists, primary care providers, and other specialists.

If you have concerns about endocrine dyscrasia or are experiencing symptoms suggestive of an endocrine disorder, it's essential to seek evaluation and management from a healthcare provider or endocrinologist. They can perform appropriate tests, provide a proper diagnosis, and recommend treatment options based on your individual circumstances.

"**Fibroadenoma of the breast**" refers to a common benign (non-cancerous) tumor that arises from the glandular and connective tissue of the breast. Fibroadenomas are typically firm, smooth, and well-defined lumps that can vary in size. They are most commonly found in women in their 20s and 30s, but they can occur at any age.

The term "coefficient" is not typically used in the context of fibroadenomas of the breast. However, if you are referring to factors or measurements associated with fibroadenomas, there are several *considerations:*

- Size: Fibroadenomas can vary in size, from less than a centimeter to several centimeters in diameter.

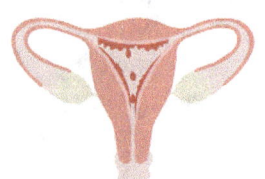

- Growth Rate: Fibroadenomas may remain stable in size or grow slowly over time.

- Appearance on Imaging: Fibroadenomas typically appear as well-defined, oval-shaped masses on imaging studies such as mammograms, ultrasound, or MRI.

- Symptoms: Fibroadenomas are usually painless, but they may cause tenderness or discomfort in some cases.

- Histology: Fibroadenomas are characterized by the presence of both glandular (epithelial) and stromal (connective tissue) components when examined under a microscope.

Diagnosis of fibroadenomas typically involves a combination of clinical evaluation, imaging studies, and sometimes biopsy to confirm the diagnosis and rule out other breast conditions, including breast cancer.

Treatment for fibroadenomas may not be necessary if they are small, stable in size, and not causing symptoms. However, some individuals may choose to have them removed surgically for reassurance or cosmetic reasons. The decision to remove a fibroadenoma depends on various factors, including the size, symptoms, and individual preferences.

If you have concerns about fibroadenomas of the breast or are experiencing breast lumps or changes, it's essential to seek evaluation and management from a healthcare provider or breast specialist. They can perform necessary tests, provide a proper diagnosis, and recommend treatment options based on your individual circumstances.

MENSTRUAL CYCLE

Beta cells are a type of cell found in the pancreas, specifically in the islets of Langerhans, and they play a crucial role in regulating blood sugar levels.

When blood sugar levels rise, such as after a meal, beta cells in the pancreas release insulin into the bloodstream. Insulin acts as a key that allows glucose (sugar) to enter cells in the body, where it can be used for energy. Additionally, insulin helps to lower blood sugar levels by promoting the storage of excess glucose in the liver and muscles as glycogen, and by inhibiting the production of glucose by the liver.

Insulin also plays a role in regulating fat metabolism and promoting the uptake of amino acids by cells for protein synthesis. Overall, insulin helps to maintain blood sugar levels within a narrow range, ensuring that cells have a steady supply of energy for proper functioning.

Deficiencies in insulin production or function can lead to diabetes mellitus, a condition characterized by high blood sugar levels. Type 1 diabetes is caused by autoimmune destruction of the beta cells, resulting in little to no insulin production. Type 2 diabetes, on the other hand, involves insulin resistance, where cells in the body do not respond effectively to insulin, leading to elevated blood sugar levels.

In summary, beta cells produce insulin, a hormone that plays a key role in regulating blood sugar levels and metabolism in the body.

In **the menstrual cycle**, various proteins play crucial roles in regulating hormonal changes, cellular processes, and tissue remodeling. Some of these proteins *include:*

- Hormones: Hormones such as estrogen and progesterone, produced by the ovaries, play key roles in regulating the menstrual cycle. These hormones help control the growth and shedding of the uterine lining during the different phases of the cycle.

- Gonadotropins: Follicle-stimulating hormone (FSH) and luteinizing hormone (LH), produced by the pituitary gland, stimulate the growth and release of eggs from the ovaries during ovulation.
- Proteins involved in tissue remodeling: During the menstrual cycle, various proteins are involved in the remodeling and shedding of the uterine lining (endometrium), including enzymes and structural proteins.

- Cytokines and growth factors: These proteins play roles in regulating inflammation, immune responses, and tissue repair processes that occur in the uterus during the menstrual cycle.

While there are many proteins involved in the menstrual cycle, there isn't a specific protein commonly referred to as "reflect protein." If you have a specific protein or aspect of the menstrual cycle in mind, please provide more context or clarify your question, and I'll be happy to assist you further.

Fibrinogen, as mentioned earlier, is a plasma protein that plays a crucial role in blood clotting. During the menstrual period, fibrinogen levels generally remain within normal ranges, unless there are underlying health conditions affecting coagulation.

The menstrual period involves the shedding of the uterine lining (endometrium) and the discharge of blood and tissue through the vagina. This process is regulated by hormonal changes, primarily involving fluctuations in estrogen and progesterone levels.

While fibrinogen itself doesn't have a direct role in the menstrual process, it's worth noting that menstrual bleeding involves a complex interplay of various factors, including the coagulation cascade. Factors involved in coagulation, such as fibrinogen, along with platelets and other clotting factors, help ensure that bleeding during menstruation is properly controlled.

However, significant abnormalities in fibrinogen levels or coagulation factors can potentially affect menstrual bleeding patterns. For example, women with bleeding disorders, such as von Willebrand disease or hemophilia, may experience heavy or prolonged menstrual bleeding due to impaired blood clotting.

If you have concerns about your menstrual bleeding patterns or suspect that you may have an underlying bleeding disorder, it's essential to consult with a healthcare provider or gynecologist for evaluation and management. They can perform appropriate tests, such as blood tests to assess coagulation factors, and provide personalized recommendations based on your individual circumstances.

The sedimentation rate, also known as the erythrocyte sedimentation rate (ESR) or "sed rate," is a blood test that measures how quickly red blood cells settle at the bottom of a tube of blood. It is a non-specific marker of inflammation and can be elevated in various inflammatory conditions, infections, and autoimmune diseases.

During the menstrual cycle, the sedimentation rate can fluctuate in response to changes in hormone levels and the inflammatory milieu within the body. However, these fluctuations are generally minor and not typically significant enough to affect clinical interpretation of the sedimentation rate test.

It's worth noting that while the menstrual cycle can influence some laboratory parameters (such as hormone levels), the sedimentation rate is primarily affected by factors related to inflammation rather than the menstrual cycle itself.

If you have concerns about your sedimentation rate or suspect that you may have an underlying inflammatory condition, it's essential to consult with a healthcare provider. They can evaluate your symptoms, medical history, and laboratory results to determine the appropriate diagnosis and management plan.

Email address
misskholeli@gmail.com

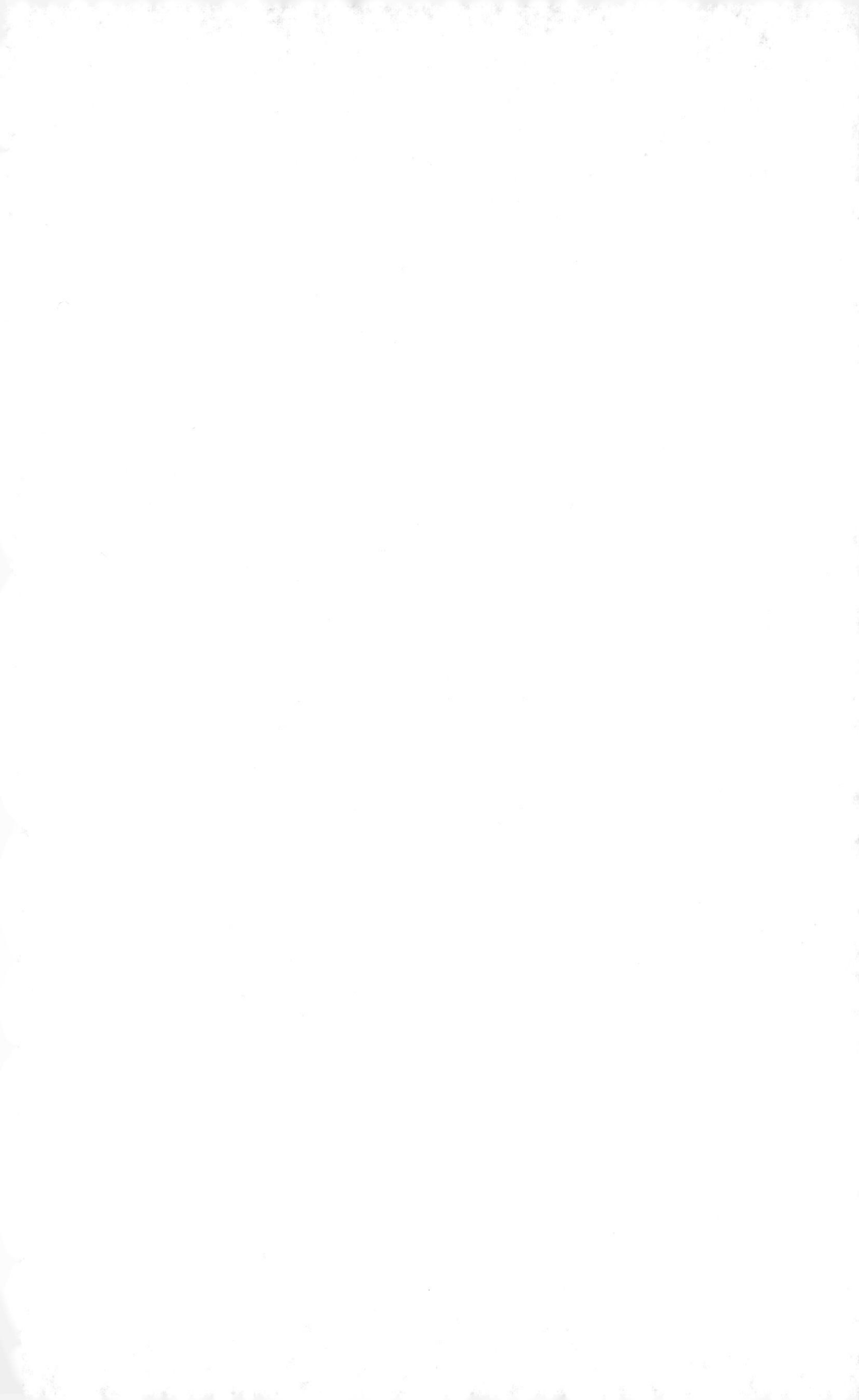